Update Gastroenterology 2004

New Developments in the Management of Benign Gastrointestinal Disorders

John Libbey Eurotext
127, avenue de la République
92120 Montrouge
Tél. : 33 (0) 1 46 73 06 60
e-mail : contact@john-libbey-eurotext.fr
http://www.john-libbey-eurotext.fr

John Libbey Eurotext Limited
42-46, High Street
Esher
Surrey
KT10 9QY
United Kingdom

© John Libbey Eurotext, 2004
ISBN : 2-7420-0538-2

Il est interdit de reproduire intégralement ou partiellement le présent ouvrage - loi du 11 mars 1957 - sans autorisation de l'éditeur ou du Centre Français du Copyright, 6 *bis*, rue Gabriel-Laumain, 75010 Paris.

Update Gastroenterology 2004

New Developments in the Management of Benign Gastrointestinal Disorders

Edited by
D.J. Gouma
G.J. Krejs
G.N.J. Tytgat
Y. Finkel

Combined EAGE, ISDS, EDS EAES and ESPGHAN
Postgraduate Course 2004
Prague, September 25-26

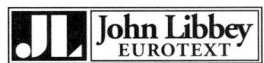

The publication of this book was made possible
thanks to the support from the NEGMA-GILD Laboratories.

Contents

I – Esophagus

How to manage the patient with oesophageal spasm
J.P. Galmiche, E.H. Metman 3

Medical treatment of achalasia
J. Tack 13

Long-term results and outcome of minimally invasive surgical treatment of GERD
B. Dallemagne 25

Management of bleeding esophageal varices: endoscopy or TIPS?
H.R. van Buuren 33

II – Bilio-pancreatic disorders

Critical appraisal of laparoscopic bile duct exploration
B. Millat 43

Management of bleeding from the papilla of Vater
D.J. Gouma 53

III – Benign GI disorders: basic concepts

Molecular biology for the gastroenterologist
P. Ferenci 59

Understanding the enteric nervous system
G.E. Boeckxstaens 69

The genetic background of gallstone formation
H.E. Wasmuth, S. Matern, F. Lammert 71

Does the COX-1/COX-2 concept still hold?
C. Hawkey 87

IV – Abdominal problems in daily practice

Free abdominal and/or retroperitoneal air. Clinical aspects
G.J. Krejs 93

Treatment of intestinal obstruction: medical aspects
J. Tack, M. Hiele, G. Coremans, L. Marchal, V. Moons 99

V – Gastrointestinal infections

Should *Helicobacter pylori* therapy be performed in all infected individuals?
P. Malfertheiner 111

The gastroenterologist looks at AIDS
J.F.W.M. Bartelsman 121

Modern management of echinococcosis
H.G. Schipper 137

Postoperative abscesses
P.B. Soeters, W. van Gemert, C.H. Dejong, J.W. Greve 155

VI – Transferring the pediatric patient to "adult" care

Celiac disease in children and adolescents
Y. Finkel 171

Celiac disease from childhood to adulthood
H. Vogelsang 175

Transition of the liver transplant recipient to adult care
D.A. Kelly 181

The IBD patient: transition from childhood to adulthood
J. Björk 193

Constipation in childhood
M.A. Benninga 201

List of contributors

Bartelsman J.F.W.M., Academic Medical Center of the University of Amsterdam, Amsterdam, The Netherlands.

Benninga M.A, Department of Paediatric Gastroenterology and Nutrition, G8-260, Emma Children's Hospital/Academic Medical Centre, Meibergdreef 9, 1195 AZ Amsterdam, The Netherlands.

Björk J., Department of Gastroenterology and Hepatology, Karolinska University Hospital, Stockholm, Sweden.

Boeckxstaens G.E., Division of Gastroenterology and Hepatology, Academic Medical Centre, Amsterdam, The Netherlands.

Coremans G., Department of Internal Medicine and Division of Gastroenterology, University Hospital Gasthuisberg, Herestraat 49, B-3000 Leuven, Belgium.

Dallemagne B., Service de Chirurgie digestive, CHC, Les Cliniques Saint-Joseph, Liège, Belgium.

Dejong C.H., Department of Surgery, Academic Hospital Maastricht, Peter Debyelaan 25, PO Box 5800, 6202 AZ Maastricht, The Netherlands.

Ferenci P., Department of Internal Medicine IV, Gastroenterology and Hepatology, University of Vienna, Allgemeines Krankenhaus, Waehringer Guertel 18-20, A 1090 Vienna, Austria.

Finkel Y., Karolinska Institute, Stockholm, Sweden.

Galmiche J.-P., Department of Gastroenterology and Hepatology, CIC INSERM and U 539, CHU, 44093 Nantes Cedex, France.

Gouma D.J., Academic Medical Center, Department of Surgery, G4-116, PO Box 22660, 1100 DD Amsterdam ZO, The Netherlands.

Greve J.W., Department of Surgery, Academic Hospital Maastricht, Peter Debyelaan 25, PO Box 5800, 6202 AZ Maastricht, The Netherlands.

Hawkey C., Wolfson Digestive Diseases Centre, University Hospital, Nottingham, NG7 2UH United Kingdom.

Hiele M., Department of Internal Medicine and Division of Gastroenterology, University Hospital Gasthuisberg, Herestraat 49, B-3000 Leuven, Belgium.

Kelly D.A., The Liver Unit, Birmingham Children's Hospital, Steelhouse Lane, Birmingham, B4 6NH, United Kingdom.

Krejs G.J., Department of Internal Medicine, University Medical Center, Auenbruggerplatz 15, A-8036 Graz, Austria.

Lammert F., Department of Medicine III, University Hospital Aachen, Aachen University (RWTH), 52074 Aachen, Germany.

Malfertheiner P., Otto-von-Guericke-University Magdeburg, Department of Gastroenterology, Hepatology and Infectious Diseases, Leipziger Str. 44, 39120 Magdeburg, Germany.

Marchal L., Department of Internal Medicine and Division of Gastroenterology, University Hospital Gasthuisberg, Herestraat 49, B-3000 Leuven, Belgium.

Matern S., Department of Medicine III, University Hospital Aachen, Aachen University (RWTH), 52074 Aachen, Germany.

Metman E.-H., Department of Gastroenterology, Hôpital Trousseau, 37044 Tours Cedex, France.

Millat B., Department of Visceral Surgery, University Hospital Saint-Éloi, 80, avenue Augustin-Fliche, 34295 Montpellier Cedex 5, France.

Moons V., Department of Internal Medicine and Division of Gastroenterology, University Hospital Gasthuisberg, Herestraat 49, B-3000 Leuven, Belgium.

Schipper H.G., Department of Internal Medicine, Division of Infectious Diseases, Tropical Medicine and AIDS, Academic Medical Center, Amsterdam, The Netherlands.

Soeters P.B., Department of Surgery, Academic Hospital, Maastricht, Peter Debyelaan 25, PO Box 5800, 6202 AZ Maastricht, The Netherlands.

Tack J., Department of Internal Medicine and Division of Gastroenterology, University Hospital Gasthuisberg, Herestraat 49, B-3000 Leuven, Belgium.

van Buuren H.R., Department of Gastroenterology and Hepatology, Erasmus Medical Centre Rotterdam, PO Box 2040 CA Rotterdam, The Netherlands.

van Gemert W., Department of Surgery, Academic Hospital Maastricht, Peter Debyelaan 25, PO Box 5800, 6202 AZ Maastricht, The Netherlands.

Vogelsang H., Department of Internal Medicine IV, Division of Gastroenterology and Hepatology, General Hospital of Vienna, Waehringer Guertel 1820, 1090 Vienna, Austria.

Wasmuth H.E., Department of Medicine III, University Hospital Aachen, Aachen University (RWTH), 52074 Aachen, Germany.

I
Esophagus

How to manage the patient with oesophageal spasm

Jean-Paul Galmiche[1], Étienne-Henry Metman[2]

[1] Department of Gastroenterology and Hepatology, CIC INSERM and U 539, CHU, 44093 Nantes cedex, France
[2] Department of Gastroenterology, Hôpital Trousseau, 37044 Tours cedex, France

Nosology and aim of therapy

The spastic oesophageal motility disorders (SOMD) comprise various abnormal manometric patterns that are typically detected in patients presenting with dysphagia and/or chest pain [1, 2]. This spectrum of conditions includes diffuse oesophageal spasm (DOS), hypersensitive lower oesophageal sphincter (HLOS) and nutcracker oesophagus. Although vigorous achalasia is also characterised by high amplitude contractions in the oesophageal body, this condition requires a similar therapeutic approach to that of achalasia in general and will not be discussed in this text. A number of manometric classifications of oesophageal motility disorders have been published [1, 3-5]. In actual fact, the pathophysiological and clinical relevance of these classifications of manometric patterns has not been established and the aetiology of SOMD remains unknown. Whereas the first studies of SOMD focused upon abnormal oesophageal body contractions (*i.e.* "spasm") as the symptom origin, there is now growing evidence that mechanisms other than disturbed motility may be involved in symptom pathogenesis [6, 7]. The role of enhanced visceral pain perception has been suggested in several observations; in particular the discordance between the symptom response (or lack of response) to various medications used in SOMD and resultant motility changes [8]. Moreover, psychiatric conditions (such as anxiety, depression, and somatisation) have been reported in a large proportion of patients with oesophageal symptoms, and chest pain of non-cardiac origin (NCCP), especially those with HLOS and nutcracker oesophagus [6]. In fact the symptoms reported by patients with SOMD may originate from both oesophageal and non-oesophageal sites as depicted by a model proposed by Clouse and Diamant [2] *(figure 1)*.

From a clinical standpoint, it is of pivotal importance to first exclude structural and metabolic disease before adopting a final diagnosis of SOMD in a patient presenting with dysphagia or chest pain. Therefore appropriate diagnostic investigations must be performed

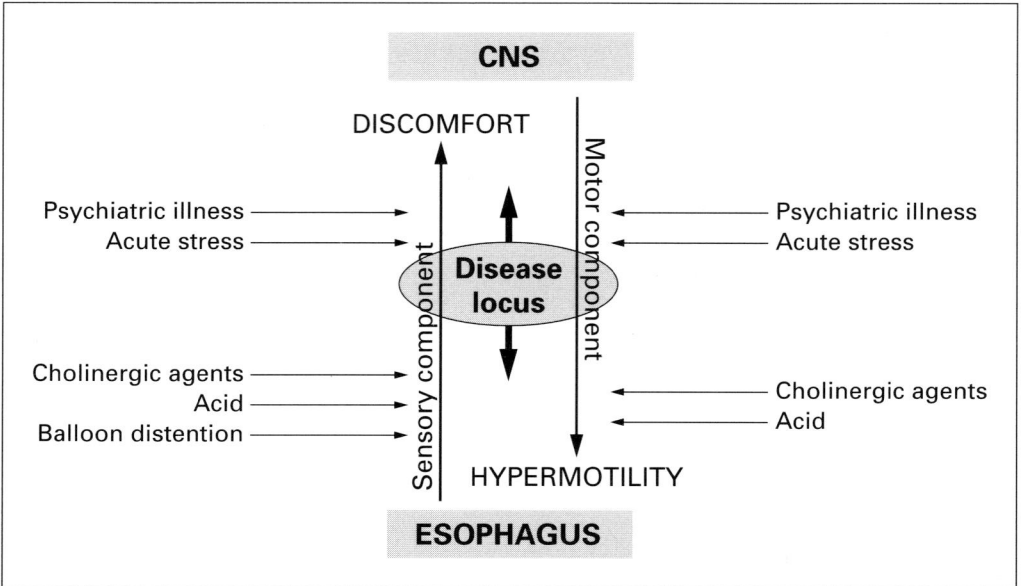

Figure 1. A working model displaying types of dysfunction found in patients with chest symptoms and spastic disorders. The location of pathology in these disorders (disease locus) is unknown and may vary within the brain-gut axis from patient to patient. Both motor and sensory components are identified, and the two processes may not be involved equally in all cases. A variety of stimuli or provoking situations are associated with or suspected of affecting the sensory and motor limbs of this model. Oesophageal hypermotility may produce symptoms directly, possibly further activate the sensory limb, or be simply a marker of the underlying process (CNS; central nervous system). Reproduced from [2] with permission from Elsevier.

and should include, as a minimum, an upper GI endoscopy in cases of dysphagia and a cardiac work-up in patients with angina-like chest pain. In addition, oesophageal manometry may contribute to the identification of a phenotype of patients with symptoms of unexplained origin and obscure mechanism.

The various paradigms proposed to explain symptoms (*i.e.* abnormal motility *versus* abnormal perception or somatisation) clearly constitute an important counterpart to the therapeutic approach. For example, drugs able to "improve" motor abnormalities may have absolutely no effect on patient symptoms. Conversely, in other cases medications may relieve symptoms without an associated effect on the motility disturbance. Finally SOMD may progress to another condition, albeit in rare cases: for example from DOS to achalasia [4]. SOMD is not typically a progressive or life-threatening illness; the sole current therapeutic aim is therefore symptom resolution.

Overview of the epidemiology and presentation of SOMD

By means of oesophageal manometry different motility patterns can be described. However, identification of these patterns is not always straightforward and overlap between various SOMDs is frequent. Various criteria have been published (including different thresholds which may affect the estimated prevalence of SOMD); the reader is invited to refer to the recent review published by Richter [1].

DOS is quite a rare disorder representing no more than 5% of all primary oesophageal motility disorders. For instance, in a series of 300 consecutive manometric studies performed in 2001 by one of the authors (EM), diagnoses of DOS and classical achalasia were established in 16 and 44 cases respectively. DOS can be detected at any stage of life; however, it is commonly identified in individuals over the age of 50. DOS is characterised by normal peristalsis that is intermittently interrupted by simultaneous contractions. Repetitive, multi-peak contractions (> 3 peaks) and spontaneous (not swallow-associated) contractions are frequently observed; the amplitude of oesophageal contractions usually exceeds 30 mmHg. Patients are hypersensitive to cholinergic and gastrinergic stimuli. Despite attempts to explain this hypersensitivity (a defect in the nitrergic inhibitory pathways has been proposed), the cause of DOS remains unknown. The barium swallow investigation is able to demonstrate tertiary activity and segmentation of the oesophagus; however, the results are variable and do not correlate with symptoms. Oesophageal 24-hour pH-monitoring must always be performed as gastroesophageal reflux is frequently present in these patients and may act as a trigger for oesophageal spasm [9]. Other provocative tests (such as balloon distension) are of less use in clinical practice, but may occasionally facilitate identification of the oesophageal origin of chest pain. 24-hour combined pH-manometry recording can increase the diagnostic yield compared to that of standard manometry and in rare instances enables the visualisation of a temporal relationship between abnormal manometric waves and episodes of chest pain [10]. However interpretation is frequently troublesome and the method that should be adopted when analysing tracings remains controversial. In some instances endoscopic ultrasonography may assist in the exclusion of a distal oesophageal obstacle responsible for motility dysfunction; in DOS it may also show an increased thickness of the muscular layer that may extend more or less proximally in the oesophagus.

The nutcracker oesophagus syndrome is defined by high amplitude contraction waves, usually greater than 180 mmHg with normal peristalsis and lower oesophageal sphincter. In contrast to achalasia and DOS, the main complaint of patients is chest pain rather than dysphagia. In fact many cases are likely to represent minor deviations from normal manometric values (2SD from normal values) with little (if any) relevance. Therefore the estimated prevalence varies highly depending on the criteria used. The HLOS is characterised by an increased resting lower oesophageal sphincter pressure (> 45 mmHg), which may occasionally be associated with incomplete oesophageal sphincter relaxation. As these two manometric patterns (nutcracker oesophagus and HLOS) may coexist, some authors have suggested that they represent a syndrome of "hypercontractile oesophagus". The results of oesophageal radiography are usually normal in both cases. Although the exact pathogenesis is unknown, exogenous factors such as stress and acid reflux are again likely to play a role *(figure 1)*.

When considering other causes of oesophageal "spasm", it must be recalled that several neurological diseases as well as systemic diseases (diabetes) can affect oesophageal motility. However, they are more frequently responsible for a *hypo*-rather than a *hyper*-contractile oesophagus. Lastly, although there is little evidence that aging affects oesophageal motility, an increased frequency of simultaneous repetitive contractions has been reported in patients over the age of 80.

Therapeutic approach of the patient with SOMD

General principles

The respective treatments of patients with DOS and those with a hypercontractile oesophagus rely on the same principles and will be discussed collectively. Asymptomatic oesophageal motility disturbances do not require any form of therapy and surveillance is usually not indicated if the patient remains symptom-free.

Reassurance of the benign nature of the disorder should always be provided, particularly to patients with episodes of angina-like chest pain. In patients with dysphagia it should be remembered that, in contrast to achalasia, associated weight loss typically does not occur. Simple measures such as drinking hot water [11] or the use of carminatives such as peppermint oil [12] may improve the symptoms of patients with a variety of motility disorders. If conditions of gastroesophageal reflux or indeed acid-related dysfunction (*i.e.* acid-sensitive oesophagus without abnormal acid exposure) are identified by pH-monitoring, they should be treated aggressively by acid suppression (proton pump inhibitors).

Treatments used for SOMD are summarised in *table I*. Drug and non-drug therapeutic approaches will be discussed; the convention being to first employ the former whilst the latter may be indicated in patients unresponsive to drug therapy.

Table I. Therapies for diffuse oesophageal spasm and hypercontractile oesophagus [1]

Reassurance
Treat underlying gastroesophageal reflux
Smooth muscle relaxants
    Nitrates
        – Sublingual Nitroglycerin 0.4 mg
        – Isosorbide dinitrate 10-30 mg twice daily
    Calcium channel blockers
        – Nifedipine 10-30 mg four times daily
        – Diltiazem 90 mg four times daily
    Anticholinergics
Psychotropic drugs
    Trazodone 100-150 mg once daily
    Imipramine 50 mg once daily
Botulinum toxin
Bougiennage
Pneumatic dilatation
Oesophageal myotomy

Drug therapy

Two comprehensive reviews concerning pharmacological therapy have been recently published [8, 13]. It should be underlined that most trials concerning SOMD are of poor methodological design; the evidence base that supports the following therapeutic guidelines is therefore relatively weak. This is mainly a result of the small samples of patients recruited and the open nature of many of the studies.

Smooth muscle relaxants

They represent the traditional pharmacological approach intended to resolve spasm. This class includes nitrate derivatives, calcium channel blockers and anticholinergics.

- **Nitrate derivatives**

These agents influence gastrointestinal motility through the stimulation of cyclic guanosine monophosphate (cGMP)-dependent pathways. To our knowledge, a placebo-controlled trial has not yet been published; however a resultant symptom improvement has been reported in several open-label studies, mainly after short-term treatment [8, 14]. In addition, the clinical use of this class of drugs is hampered by the relatively frequent occurrence of side effects (such as headache) and the theoretical risk of the promotion or aggravation of gastroesophageal reflux.

- **Calcium-channel blockers**

Although many compounds are available in this pharmacological class, experience of their use in SOMD is mainly limited to the first generation of calcium-channel blockers. Data regarding their long-term efficacy is also scarce. In a 14-week double-blind placebo-controlled cross-over trial conducted in patients with nutcracker oesophagus, nifedipine (10-30 mg tid) was found to have no effect on symptoms despite a significant reduction in contraction amplitude [15]. In contrast, diltiazem was found to ameliorate symptoms in nutcracker oesophagus by Cattau *et al.* [16], but not in DOS by Drenth *et al.* [17]. Despite these disappointing results, some patients seem to be really improved by calcium blockers on long-term follow up as suggested by several open-label studies (for review see [8]). Long-acting compounds are more appropriate for the treatment of chest pain.

- **Anticholinergics**

These agents (*e.g.* L-hyoscyamine) are known to reduce the amplitude of distal oesophageal peristalsis and to attenuate the pain induced by balloon distension in healthy subjects. The role of more selective muscarinic receptor antagonists such as the M1 antagonist pirenzepin remains to be evaluated as their pharmacological action results in an increased propagation of peristaltic waves accompanied by a reduction in contraction amplitude.

Psychotropic drugs

It has been convincingly established that low-dose antidepressant medications can ameliorate both pain and discomfort in patients with a variety of oesophageal motility disorders without affecting oesophageal motility [18, 19]. It is likely that this analgesic effect is independent of an effect on mood. Again these studies emphasise the role of hypersensitivity and/or increased reactivity to various stresses that have been consistently reported in several studies conducted in patients with NCCP, irrespective of motility pattern.

Trazodone (100-150 mg/day) has been shown to be effective in various non-specific motility disorders associated with chest pain [20] and a recent retrospective analysis by Prakash and Clouse [21] suggests that treatment remains effective for up to three years. Similarly **imipramine** (50 mg nocte) was found to be superior to a placebo in patients with NCCP irrespective of oesophageal motility disturbances [22]. Other uncontrolled observations have also suggested that different combinations of **psychotherapy and trazodone or clomipramine** may be beneficial in patients with DOS [8].

Recently developed drug therapies

Botulinum toxin (Botox) inhibits the calcium-dependent release of acetylcholine from cholinergic nerve terminals. As Botox injections into the lower oesophageal sphincter have been shown to effectively relieve dysphagia and pain in more than 80% of achalasia patients, some researchers [23, 24] have attempted to employ this form of therapy in patients with SOMD that are not responsive to the aforementioned traditional drug approaches. Experience in SOMD is however much more limited than in achalasia. Miller *et al.* [24] reported a favourable effect of Botox in approximately 70% of 29 patients with various SOMD. In our experience, out of 13 patients treated with Botox for SOMD, 8% failed to respond, 54% had a sustained remission of several months (a mean of 20 months) whilst the remainder relapsed after six to eight months and therefore needing two or even three injections to maintain the beneficial effect. Different injection protocols have been applied; for example, Storr *et al.* [13] have used multiple injections at different sites in the oesophageal body of nine DOS patients. Although these preliminary reports are encouraging, a controlled trial is yet to be published.

Nitric oxide donors. Nitric oxide (NO) is recognised as the most important transmitter of the non-adrenergic, non-cholinergic inhibitory neural pathways. The enzyme responsible for the production of NO (NO-synthase) uses L-arginine as a substrate for this synthesis. Recently several attempts have been made to influence oesophageal motility by the administration of **L-arginine** either orally or intravenously. In a preliminary randomised placebo-controlled trail of eight patients with chest pain and oesophageal motor disorders, Bortolotti *et al.* [25] observed a significant reduction in symptoms after six weeks of oral L-arginine administration. This treatment was well tolerated; however, due to the small size of the trial, such research needs to be reproduced and verified.

Sildenafil is a phosphodiesterase type-5 inhibitor which results in accumulation of NO stimulated cGMP. Sildenafil has been shown to inhibit the oesophageal contractile activity in both healthy human subjects and achalasia patients [26, 27]. In a recent study conducted in eleven patients with a variety of oesophageal motility disorders, sildenafil improved manometric parameters in nine patients, but symptoms in only four individuals *(table II)*. Two patients discontinued the treatment on account of side effects.

Table II. Effects of sildenafil in four SOMD patients with symptomatic improvement when treated on a prn basis

Sex	Age	Symptoms	Manometric features before sildenafil	1 h after sildenafil 50 mg	Comments
F	57	Dysphagia	Hypertensive LOS: 80 mm Hg	16 mm Hg	Under 25 mg sildenafil no symptoms > 4 months No side effects Nifedipine causes dizziness
F	54	Dysphagia and heartburn	Corpus: segm, simult, contr. 70 mm Hg LOS 76 mm Hg	No obvious contraction 10 mm Hg	10 days treatment Dysphagia improved However sleep disturbances
F	36	Dysphagia	Nutcracker: corpus ampl. up to 160 mm Hg Duration of pressure wave > 9 s LOS post-deglutitive > 120 mm Hg	60 mm Hg Below 4 s LOS 20 mm Hg	1 week treatment Dysphagia improved However feeling of tightness in the chest at night
F	41	Dysphagia, heartburn	Nutcracker: post-deglut. LOS 65 mm Hg Corpus amplitudes up to 160 mm Hg	Below 20 mm Hg No corpus motility detectable	> 4 weeks Dysphagia and heartburn improved Better effect than diltiazem

Adapted from Eherer *et al.* [28].

In summary, there is a credible rationale for research into the use of NO donors for the treatment of patients with SOMD. However, agents that are both more effective and better tolerated are needed; larger placebo-controlled trials would be required before such compounds are adopted in clinical practice.

Selective serotonine reuptake inhibitors (SSRIs). Following the finding that the administration of trazodone and imipramine may benefit patients with NCCP, a recent placebo-controlled trial has evaluated the effect of the SSRI **sertraline** (50 mg to 200 mg) in this group of patients. Although a significant reduction in pain score was reported, information on motility function was not available from this trial [29]. Side effects (nausea, decreased libido, delayed ejaculation and restlessness) occurred in 27% of patients.

Beside antidepressants there is a host of potential compounds likely to be able to reduce the enhanced visceral perception or hyperalgesia observed in patients with SOMD. These include **somatostatin analogues**, **5HT$_3$ antagonists**, **theophylline** [30] **and the kappa-opioid receptor agonist (fedotozine)**. However as yet none of them has reached the evidential threshold necessary to be applied clinically.

Non-drug therapy

Dilatation

This treatment is generally proposed following failure of different medications. Static dilatation (bougiennage) is usually ineffective [1] whereas pneumatic dilatation of the cardia is of greatest efficacy, particularly in patients with predominant symptoms of dysphagia [31, 32]. In our experience, pneumatic dilatation was necessary in approximately 1/3 of patients with SOMD and was found to improve symptoms in 3/4 of them. However, as with Botulinum toxin treatment, this intervention needs to be repeated in order to maintain remission. It is a relatively safe procedure and even rare complications such as perforation can be treated conservatively with excellent results.

Surgical myotomy

In some patients with refractory symptoms, a long myotomy can be proposed and success rates exceeding 50% have been reported [33, 34]. However long-term surgical results for pain management do not appear promising [35]. This treatment was applied to eight out of our 31 SOMD patients. No mortality was observed and three individuals remained completely or partially improved after an average follow-up period of 34 months. The remaining five patients suffered relapses after an average interval of 40 months. In line with this experience and existing literature, the use of myotomy in the treatment of SOMD should be reserved for patients whose quality of life is profoundly affected by severe symptoms which are refractory to other treatments and can be reliably linked to motor abnormalities. In these difficult cases, preoperative endoscopic ultrasonography may be valuable in the objective assessment of the level of muscular thickening and therefore the extent of the myotomy to be performed.

In conclusion, the treatment of patients with SOMD remains a challenging issue. Approximately half of patients find that their symptoms are improved by traditional drug approaches; however tachyphylaxis frequently occurs. Gastroesophageal reflux should always be considered and, if present, treated aggressively by proton pump inhibitors. Many patients who either fail to respond to or do not require drug therapy are helped by pneumatic dilatation or injections of botulinum toxin; however, these procedures need to be repeated to maintain remission. Ultimately, surgical myotomy must be reserved for the group of highly selected patients with severe chest pain which fails to respond to previous measures.

References

1. Richter JE. Oesophageal motility disorders. *Lancet* 2001; 358: 823-8.
2. Clouse RE, Diamant NE. Esophageal motor and sensory function and motor disorders of the esophagus. In: Feldman M, Friedman LS, Sleisenger MH, eds. *Gastrointestinal and liver disease: pathophysiology, diagnosis, management*, 7th ed. Philadelphia: W.B. Saunders, 2002 (volume 1): 561-98.
3. Cohen S. Motor disorders of the esophagus. *N Engl J Med* 1979; 301: 186-92.
4. Vantrappen G, Janssens H, Hellemans J, Coremans G. Achalasia, diffuse esophageal spasm, and related motility disorders. *Gastroenterology* 1979; 76: 450-7.

5. Spechler SJ, Castell DO. Classification of oesophageal motility abnormalities. *Gut* 2001; 49: 145-51.
6. Song CW, Lee SJ, Jeen YT, Chun HJ, Um SH, Kim CD, et al. Inconsistent association of esophageal symptoms, psychometric abnormalities and dysmotility. *Am J Gastroenterol* 2001; 96: 2312-6.
7. Prakash C, Clouse RE. Esophageal motor disorders. *Curr Opin Gastroenterol* 2002; 18: 545-63.
8. Achem SR. Treatment of spastic esophageal motility disorders. *Gastroenterol Clin North Am* 2004; 33: 107-24.
9. Börjesson M, Pilhall M, Rolny P, Mannheimer C. Gastroesophageal acid reflux in patients with nutcracker esophagus. *Scand J Gastroenterol* 2001; 36: 916-20.
10. Barham CP, Gotley DC, Fowler A, Mills A, Alderson D. Diffuse esophageal spasm: diagnosis by ambulatory 24 hour manometry. *Gut* 1997; 41: 151-5.
11. Triadafilopoulos G, Tsang HP, Segall GM. Hot water swallows improve symptoms and accelerate esophageal clearance in esophageal motility disorders. *J Clin Gastroenterol* 1998; 26: 239-44.
12. Pimentel M, Bonorris GG, Chow EJ, Lin HC. Peppermint oil improves the manometric findings in diffuse esophageal spasm. *J Clin Gastroenterol* 2001; 33: 27-31.
13. Storr M, Allescher HD, Classen M. Current concepts on pathophysiology diagnosis and treatment of diffuse esophageal spasm. *Drugs* 2001; 61: 579-91.
14. Mellow MH. Effect of isosorbide and hydralazine in painful primary esophageal motility disorders. *Gastroenterology* 1982; 83: 364-70.
15. Richter JE, Dalton CB, Bradley LA, Castell DO. Oral nifedipine in the treatment of noncardiac chest pain in patients with the nutcracker esophagus. *Gastroenterology* 1987; 93: 21-8.
16. Cattau El Jr, Castell DO, Johnson DA, Spurling TJ, Hirszel R, Chobanian SI, et al. Diltiazem therapy for symptoms associated with nutcracker esophagus. *Am J Gastroenterol* 1991; 86: 272-6.
17. Drenth JP, Bos LP, Engels LG. Efficacy of diltiazem in the treatment of diffuse oesophageal spasm. *Aliment Pharmacol Ther* 1990; 4: 411-6.
18. Handa M, Mine K, Yamamoto H, Hayashi H, Tsuchida O, Kanazawa F, Kubo C. Antidepressant treatment of patients with diffuse esophageal spasm: a psychosomatic approach. *J Clin Gastroenterol* 1999; 28: 228-32.
19. Clouse RE. Antidepressants for functional gastrointestinal syndromes. *Dig Dis Sci* 1994; 39: 2352-63.
20. Clouse RE, Lustman PJ, Eckert TC, Ferney DM, Griffith LS. Low-dose trazodone for symptomatic patients with esophageal contraction abnormalities. A double-blind, placebo-controlled trial. *Gastroenterology* 1987; 92: 1027-36.
21. Prakash C, Clouse RE. Long-term outcome from tricyclic antidepressant treatment of functional chest pain. *Dig Dis Sci* 1999; 44: 2373-9.
22. Cannon RO 3rd, Quyyumi AA, Mincemoyer R, Stine AM, Gracely RH, Smith WB, Geraci MF, Black BC, Uhde TW, Waclawiw MA. Imipramine in patients with chest pain despite normal coronary angiograms. *N Engl J Med* 1994; 330: 1411-7.
23. Storr M, Allescher HD, Rosch T. Treatment of symptomatic diffuse esophageal spasm by endoscopic injections of botulinum toxin: a prospective study with long term follow-up. *Gastrointest Endosc* 2001; 54: 754-9.
24. Miller LS, Pullela SV, Parkman HP, Schiano TD, Cassidy MJ, Cohen S, Fisher RS. Treatment of chest pain in patients with noncardiac, nonreflux, nonachalasia spastic esophageal motor disorders using botulinum toxin injection into the gastroesophageal junction. *Am J Gastroenterol* 2002; 97: 1640-6.
25. Bortolotti M, Brunelli F, Sarti P, Miglioli M. Clinical and manometric effects of L-arginine in patients with chest pain and oesophageal motor disorders. *Ital J Gastroenterol Hepatol* 1997; 29: 320-4.
26. Bortolotti M, Mari C, Lopilato C, Porrazzo G, Miglioki M. Effects of sildenafil on esophageal motility of patients with idiopathic achalasia. *Gastroenterology* 2000; 118: 253-7.
27. Bortolotti M, Mari C, Giovannini M, Pinna S, Miglioli M. Effects of sildenafil on esophageal motility of normal subjects. *Dig Dis Sci* 2001; 46: 2301-6.

28. Eherer AJ, Schwetz I, Hammer HF, Petnehazy T, Scheidl SJ, Weber K, Krejs GJ. Effect of sildenafil on oesophageal motor function in healthy subjects and patients with oesophageal motor disorders. *Gut* 2002; 50: 758-64.
29. Varia I, Logue E, O'Connor C, Newby K, Wagner R, Davenport C, Rathey K, Krishnan KR. Randomized trial of sertraline in patients with unexplained chest pain of noncardiac origin. *Am Heart J* 2000; 140: 67-72.
30. Rao SSC, Mudipalli RS, Mujica V, Utech GL, Zhao X, Conklin JL. An open-label trial of theophylline for functional chest pain. *Dig Dis Sci* 2002; 47: 2763-8.
31. Vantrappen G, Hellemans J. Treatment of achalasia and related motor disorders. *Gastroenterology* 1980; 79: 144-54.
32. Irving JD, Owen WJ, McCullagh M, Keighley A, Anggiansah A. Management of diffuse esophageal spasm with balloon dilatation. *Gastrointest Radiol* 1992; 17: 189-92.
33. Horton ML, Goff JS. Surgical treatment of nutcracker esophagus. *Dig Dis Sci* 1986; 31: 878-83.
34. Eypasch EP, DeMeester TR, Klingman RR, Stein HJ. Physiologic assessment and surgical management of diffuse esophageal spasm. *J Thorac Cardiovasc Surg* 1992: 104: 859-69.
35. Ellis FH Jr. Long esophagomyotomy for diffuse esophageal spasm and related disorders: an historical overview. *Dis Esophagus* 1998; 11: 210-4.

Medical treatment of achalasia

Jan Tack

Department of Internal Medicine, Division of Gastroenterology, University Hospital Gasthuisberg, Catholic University of Leuven, Leuven, Belgium

Achalasia

Most symptoms and complications of achalasia are due to retention of food and fluid in the esophagus, as a result of defective relaxation of an often hypertensive lower esophageal sphincter, together with loss of propulsive peristalsis in the esophageal body [1-3]. This is caused by the loss of intrinsic inhibitory neurons in the lower esophageal sphincter, while intrinsic excitatory (cholinergic) neurons are preserved [4, 5]. The current treatment of achalasia and related motor disorders is at best palliative. It is still impossible to restore the disordered motility of the achalatic esophagus to normal. Therefore, treatment should aim to improve esophageal emptying by decreasing the resistance at the cardia sufficiently to allow easy aboral flow, thereby taking care that the sphincter continues to present a pressure barrier to prevent free gastro-esophageal reflux. Non-surgical means of diminishing the resistance at the cardia consist of drugs, forceful dilatations of the cardia, and endoscopic injection of botulinum toxin.

Drug treatment

Several pharmacological agents have been used in an attempt to decrease the lower esophageal sphincter pressure in patients with achalasia. Most studies, however, have evaluated only relatively short-term effects, often in patients with only mild or moderate degrees of achalasia. There are very few studies devoted to the long-term evaluation of medical therapy for achalasia, or to the comparison of drug therapy with other means of treatment.

Earlier therapeutic trials with anticholinergic agents and adrenergic blockers failed to show a substantial benefit [6-8]. Cimetropium bromide, an anticholinergic, was shown to be able to reduce the lower esophageal sphincter pressure significantly and accelerate esophageal transit in patients with achalasia [9]. One study reported a decrease in lower esophageal sphincter pressure in patients with achalasia administered high doses of loperamide [10]. No data on clinical use of these drugs have been published so far.

In the eighties, nitrates and calcium antagonists were found to decrease the lower esophageal sphincter pressure and they have been used in an attempt to relieve achalasia symptoms.

Calcium channel blockers

Calcium entry blockers have a relaxant effect on vascular and gastrointestinal smooth muscle. Nifedipine (10-20 mg) has been shown to reduce significantly the lower esophageal sphincter resting pressure (maximum reduction 56%) and, at higher doses, the amplitude of esophageal body contractions (maximum reduction 35%) in healthy volunteers [11-13].

Administration of 10-20 mg nifedipine in achalasia patients significantly reduces the lower esophageal sphincter pressure (maximum reduction 47%) [14, 15]. In a dose of 10 to 20 mg given sublingually before each meal, nifedipine improved the symptoms of dysphagia in 14 out of 20 patients with mild to moderate achalasia (stage I and II according to Adam's criteria) during a follow-up period of 6 to 18 months [14]. In a non-randomized follow-up study, treatment with nifedipine, 10-20 mg sublingual 30 minutes before each meal, was compared with pneumatic dilatation in a randomized trial in 30 patients. Both treatments proved equally effective: excellent or good clinical results were observed in 75% of dilated patients and 77% of nifedipine treated patients [16]. Again, this trial was carried out in patients with mild to moderate achalasia. In another study (a cross-over trial with nitrates), 15 patients with achalasia were treated with nifedipine, 20 mg sublingual before the meal [15]. This study also included nine patients with a dilated esophagus (stage III). Only eight patients (53%) noted relief of dysphagia by nifedipine.

In a double-blind placebo-controlled study, nifedipine 10-30 mg sublingual in ten achalasia patients was found to significantly reduce the frequency of dysphagia, but substantial symptoms remained present during drug therapy [17]. Chronic nifedipine treatment decreased the lower esophageal sphincter pressure only moderately (by 28%, still leaving lower esophageal sphincter pressures of 30 to 35 mm Hg) while the radionuclide measurement of esophageal emptying remained unchanged [17]. Side effects, such as peripheral edema, headache, flushing and hypotension, were relatively common, but did not usually require discontinuation of the drug.

Finally, a double-blind crossover study with oral nifedipine (20 mg orally one hour before each meal), verapamil (160 mg orally one hour before each meal) and placebo in eight patients with stage II achalasia failed to demonstrate statistically significant differences in the overall clinical symptomatology with any of the drugs [18]. This study used oral instead of sublingual nifedipine, but adequate nifedipine plasma levels were documented. The effect of diltiazem (120 mg orally) on lower esophageal sphincter pressure and on symptoms in patients with achalasia (60 to 90 mg orally QID) was only marginal [19].

Nitrates

Nitrates have a relaxant effect on smooth muscle of a variety of species and tissues, including the gastrointestinal tract in man. Early radiographic studies demonstrated a relaxation of the cardia of achalasia patients in response to nitrite inhalation or sublingual nitroglycerin [20-22]. However, this effect was short-lived (4 to 30 minutes) and associated with several side-effects.

The long-acting form of nitroglycerin, isosorbide dinitrate, was found to reduce the mean lower esophageal sphincter pressure by 66% in patients with achalasia, for at least 60 minutes [15, 23]. In a dose of 5 mg given sublingually before each meal, isosorbide dinitrate improved symptoms of dysphagia in 19 of 23 patients during a follow-up period of 2 to 19 months, but side effects (mainly headaches) were very common (8/24 patients) [15].

A randomized cross-over study compared the effect of a two-week treatment of isosorbide dinitrate 5 mg sublingually before meals with that of nifedipine 20 mg in 15 patients with achalasia [15]. Isosorbide dinitrate induced a more pronounced acute reduction in lower esophageal sphincter pressure when compared with nifedipine (63% *versus* 47%), resulted in a larger degree of subjective improvement (thirteen *versus* eight patients), but had also a higher rate of side effects (six *versus* two patients). However, radionuclide measurement of esophageal emptying still demonstrated considerable esophageal retention in four patients with subjective benefit. Therapeutic failure necessitated pneumatic dilatation in six of the fifteen patients.

Studies investigating the medical treatment of achalasia have yielded conflicting results. The apparent differences may rely mainly on patient selection, and on outcome measures. Studies in patients without a dilated esophagus seem to yield better results, and patients with marked esophageal dilatation may respond less well to pharmacological treatment. It seems that pharmacological treatment has at least some clinical efficacy in diminishing symptoms of dysphagia: even negative studies report improved symptoms in a subset of patients. However, the response is considerably less good, when other symptom criteria than dysphagia are taken into account.

In view of the limitations of the currently available drug therapy (limited reduction in lower esophageal sphincter pressure, frequent failure to improve esophageal emptying rate, high failure rate due to insufficient potency, side effects or progression of the disease), it seems hard to justify their life-long use when other treatment modalities, *i.e.* pneumatic dilatation or surgery, result in excellent or good long-term results in over 80% of the patients. It seems reasonable, therefore, to restrict drug therapy to the following indications: i) as a temporary measure until more definitive treatment is performed, ii) as an adjuvant therapy for patients in whom dilatation or surgery was only partially successful, and iii) as a palliative therapy in patients with an unacceptably high risk for more invasive therapy and with no response to botulinum toxin. In these instances, nifedipine (10-20 mg) or isosorbide dinitrate (5 mg) sublingually before each meal seems appropriate. Transcutaneous nerve stimulation has recently been reported to relieve dysphagia in a small number of patients with achalasia, but obviously requires further studies [24, 25].

Pneumatic dilatation

Pneumatic dilatation is still the most effective non-surgical treatment modality in achalasia. Although details of the dilatation procedure vary from institution to institution, they all aim at mechanical disruption of the muscle fibers at the esophago-gastric junction. There is some controversy about the frequency at which dilatation should be repeated, about the parameters of dilatation that should be used, and whether or not the procedure should be carried out under general anesthesia. Several types of dilators have been proposed. The most frequently used type is the Rigiflex dilator balloon, a polyurethane balloon which is positioned at the lower esophageal sphincter over an (endoscopically positioned) guide wire and inflated to a diameter of 3.0, 3.5 or 4.0 cm. In addition, endoscopic pneumatic dilators have become available, which allow placement across the gastroesophageal junction under direct vision. Endoscopically guided pneumatic dilatation, in

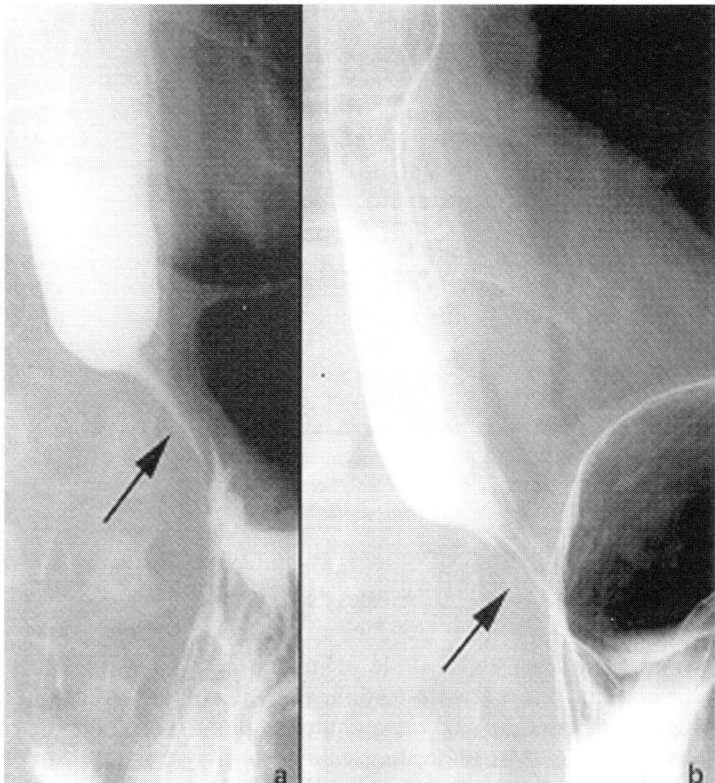

Figure 1. Radiological picture of achalasia (a) before and (b) after pneumatic dilatation.

the absence of fluoroscopic control, seems to be both safe and efficient [31-36]. Depending on the clinical efficacy and the residual sphincter pressure, several dilatation sessions (classically up to three) with increasing balloon diameters can be performed [26-41]. Only few studies assessed the effect of clinical and dilatation parameters on outcome in patients undergoing pneumatic dilatation for achalasia. In one prospective study, esophageal transit, symptoms, esophageal transit and diameter did not predict the symptomatic response to pneumatic dilatation [40]. Furthermore, the size of the dilator, the frequency of the dilatation and the duration of inflation of the balloon had no effect on the success of pneumatic dilatation. Follow-up studies have indicated that the best predictor for a long-term remission is a residual sphincter pressure below 10 mm Hg [42].

In case of a tortuous and severely dilated esophagus, these dilators may be difficult to pass through the cardia. In these cases, prior to dilatation, the patient swallows a mercury-filled latex bag to which a nylon string is attached. As soon as the mercury-filled bag has passed into small intestine, the nylon wire can be used as a guide wire. At the start of each dilatation session, a metal wire with an eye at the end is threaded over the nylon string into the stomach to provide a rigid guide for the introduction of the dilator.

Pneumatic dilatation yields good to excellent results in 70-80% of patients *(table I)*, especially in patients over 45 years old, in patients with a longer standing history (> five years of symptoms) and in patients with a slightly dilated esophagus. However, it seems that the longer term outcome is less favorable, and recurrence is seen in the majority of patients when followed over several years *(table I)*.

Table I. Long-term response to pneumatic dilatation in achalasia

Study	N	Follow-up (years)	Success rate (%)
Olsen, 1951	452	4-16	69
Sanderson, 1970	313	2.5	65
Burnett, 1970	48	2.5	70
Wienbeck, 1975	21	3.2	81
Heimlich, 1978	25	2.5	84
Vantrappen, 1980	403	7.8	77
Wevers, 1985	184	4.5	70
Eckardt, 1992	54	4	50
Eckardt, 1997	67	5	44
Torbey, 1999	47	6.8	36
Allescher, 2001	37	4	35
West, 2002	127	12	40

Contra-indications to pneumatic dilatations are: i) inability of the patient to cooperate because of age, such as in small children, or the presence of psychosis, ii) the inability to rule out an organic stenosis, iii) the presence of lesions at the cardia or stomach, which makes surgery mandatory, and iv) the presence of an epiphrenic diverticulum, which increases the risk of perforation. Old age, a poor cardiopulmonary condition, a grossly dilated and sigmoid-shaped esophagus or previous cardiomyotomy do not constitute contra-indications for pneumatic dilatation. The most important complication of pneumatic dilatation is an esophageal perforation, which is reported in 2 to 6% of the patients. In general these can be managed conservatively with no foods orally and intravenous antibiotics until healing of the lesion, usually within 7 to 14 days. However, the litterature does report a mortality of 0.3% in case of perforation. Risk factors for perforation are a high intra-balloon pressure, increasing diameter of the balloon, duration of the dilatation and vigorous type of achalasia. The most important long-term complication is gastroesophageal reflux, which has been reported to occur in 0 to 30%. When no clinical benefit is obtained after three to four dilatations, surgery should be considered.

The major immediate complication of dilatation is perforation at the lower end of the esophagus, which occurs in 1-5% of patients according to the literature. In our experience, perforation occurred in 2.6%. The risk of perforation is higher if patients had had previous dilatations or when inflation pressures of above 11 psi are used [43]. Despite widely held opinion to the contrary, perforation after pneumatic dilatation can be treated safely and effectively by parenteral nutrition, broad-spectrum antibiotics and continuous esophageal aspiration, provided that perforation is recognized early and, and that the patient remained fasted [30]. The most troublesome late complication after forceful dilatation is reflux esophagitis and reflux-induced stricture formation. In our experience, stricture formation was seen in only 0.7% of the patients.

Injection of botulinum toxin

Botulinum toxin blocks the presynaptic release of acetylcholine at the neuromuscular junction. Animal data have indicated that intrasphincteric injection of botulinum toxin is able to lower esophageal sphincter pressure [44]. In subsequent studies, it was established that intrasphincteric administration of botulinum toxin is able to decrease the lower esophageal sphincter pressure in patients with achalasia [45, 46]. In a double-blind, placebo-controlled trial, it was shown that intrasphincteric injection of botulinum toxin in patients with achalasia is able to decrease manometric abnormalities and to provide a significant improvement in symptoms in about two-thirds of the patients [44-49]. Higher success rates are seen in patients over 50 years of age and in patients with vigorous achalasia.

Because of its simplicity, injection of botulinum toxin gained rapid acceptance as a treatment for achalasia. However, although the initial rate of symptomatic benefit may be comparable to that of pneumatic dilatations, the effect wears off quickly in many patients, and a prolonged response (six-twelve months) is obtained in only about 50% of the patients

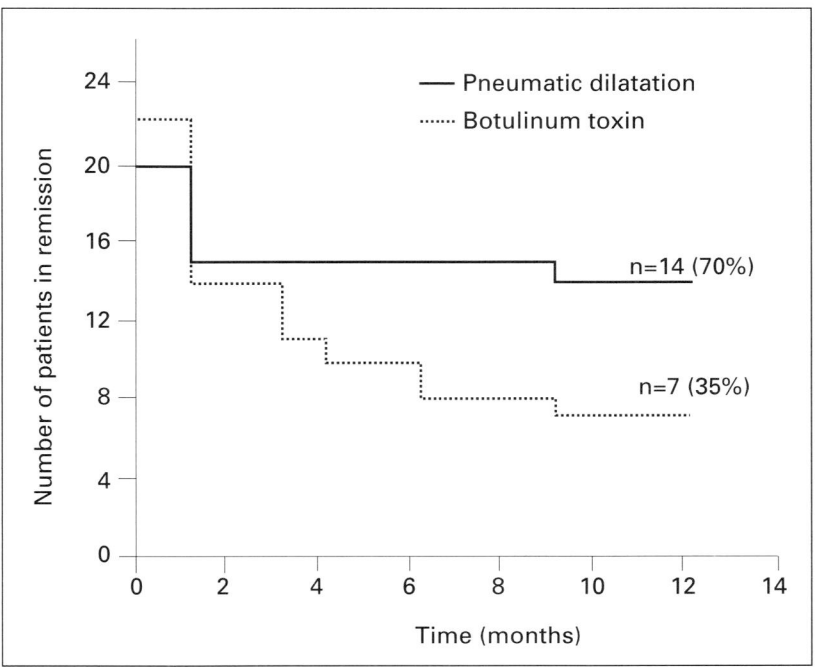

Figure 2. Responses to pneumatic dilatation and botulinum toxin injection in a randomized controlled trial. Adapted from Vaezi *et al.*, 1999.

[46, 47]. These usually respond to a second injection. Nevertheless, studies comparing botulinum toxin injection to pneumatic dilatation generally shows more favorable results with pneumatic dilatation *(table II)* [48, 49].

Choice of therapy

The Heller myotomy procedure yields good results in 63-95% of the patients [50-58]. A full discussion of surgical treatment can be found in the chapter on "Surgical treatment of achalasia". Most literature data comparing surgical therapy and pneumatic dilatation are based on retrospective studies [59-63]. In a retrospective analysis, comparing the effect of surgery with pneumatic dilatation, the overall success rate of pneumatic dilatation was comparable to that of surgery (88% *versus* 89%). Symptomatic relief was comparable in both groups, but heartburn occurred more frequently following myotomy [1]. The total cost for initial esophagomyotomy was calculated to be 2.4 times higher than for initial pneumatic dilatation [56, 61]. The only prospective study published so far yielded excellent or good long-term results in 95% of patients after myotomy, compared with 65% after dilatation, which is, however, an abnormally low success rate for pneumatic dilatations in comparison to results reported by other groups [62].

Table II. Comparison between pneumatic dilatation and botulinum toxin injection in achalasia

Study	N	Follow-up	Retreatment	Outcome
Annese, 1996	16	12 months	Yes	Equal
Vaezi, 1999	42	12 months	Yes (once)	Pneumatic dilatation superior
Muehldorfer, 1999	24	30 months	No	Pneumatic dilatation superior
Prakash, 1999 (not randomized)	68	24 months	Yes	Equal
Mikaeli, 2001	40	12 months	Yes	Pneumatic dilatation superior
Ghoshal, 2001	14	8 months	No	Pneumatic dilatation superior
Allescher, 2001	37	48 months	Yes	Equal at 12 months. Dilatation superior at 24 and 48 months

The advantages of pneumatic dilatations are that it is a low cost, safe procedure which can be performed on an out-patient basis. The progress in minimally invasive surgery has strongly enhanced the attractivity of the surgical approach to achalasia. As both are techniques with good longer-term results, the expertise of the surgeon with myotomy or of the endoscopist with dilatation seems a reasonable base to determine the choice between both for a particular patient. In our center, we still use pneumatic dilatation as a primary approach, as it seems easier to operate on patients who did not respond to pneumatic dilatation than to dilate patients who did not respond to a Heller myotomy. Due to its less invasive nature and low risk compared to other therapies, the treatment of achalasia using botulinum toxin appears to be an interesting alternative in patients who are not suitable for or who refuse conventional therapy.

Table III. Comparison between pneumatic dilatation and myotomy in achalasia

Author	% response to dilatation	% response to myotomy
Bennett, 1970	81	69
Spitzer, 1973	94	93
Csendes, 1974/5	83	95
Arvanitakis, 1975	67	91
Yon, 1975	46	85
Okike, 1979	81	94
Csendes, 1981	60	100

References

1. Vantrappen G, Van Goidsenhoven GE, Verbeke S, Van Den Berghe G, Vandenbroucke J. Manometric studies in achalasia of the cardia, before and after pneumatic dilatations. *Gastroenterology* 1963; 45; 317-25.
2. Vantrappen G, Janssens J, Hellemans J, Coremans G. Achalasia, diffuse esophageal spasm, and related motility disorders. *Gastroenterology* 1979; 76; 450.
3. Vantrappen G, Hellemans J. Achalasia. In: Vantrappen G, Hellemans J, eds. *Diseases of the oesophagus*. Berlin, Heidelberg, New York: Springer-Verlag, 1975; 287-354.
4. Mearin F, Mourelle M, Guarner F, Salas A, Riveros-Moreno V, Moncada S, Malagelada JR. Patients with achalasia lack nitric oxide synthase in the gastro-oesophageal junction. *Eur J Clin Invest* 1993; 23: 724-8.
5. Holloway RH, Dodds WJ, Helm JF, Hogan WJ, Dent J, Arndorfer RC. Integrity of cholinergic innervation to the lower esophageal sphincter in achalasia. *Gastroenterology* 1986; 90: 924.
6. Christensen J. Effects of drugs on esophageal motility. *Arch Intern Med* 1976; 136; 532-7.
7. Lobis JB, Fischer RS. Anticholinergic therapy for achalasia. A controlled study. *Gastroenterology* 1976; 70: 976.
8. Nickerson M, Call LS. Treatment of cardiospasm with adrenergic blockade. *Am J Med* 1957; 11; 123-7.
9. Marzio L, Grossi L, DeLaurentis MF, Cennamo L, Lapenna D, Cucurullo F. Effect of cimetropium bromide on esophageal motility and transit in patients affected by primary achalasia. *Dig Dis Sci* 1994; 39: 1389-94.
10. Penagini, Bartesaghi B, Negri G, Bianchi PA. Effect of loperamide on lower oesophageal sphincter pressure in idiopathic achalasia. *Scand J Gastroenterol* 1994; 29: 1057-60.
11. Blackwell JN, Holt S, Heading RC. Effect of nifedipine on oesophageal motility and gastric emptying. *Digestion* 1981; 21; 50-6.
12. Hongo M, Traube M, McAllister RG, McCallum RW. Effects of nifedipine on esophageal motor function in humans: Correlation with plasma nifedipine concentration. *Gastroenterology* 1984; 84: 8-12.
13. Weiser HF, Lepsien G, Golenhofen K, Siewert R. Clinical and experimental studies on the effect of nifedipine on smooth muscle of the oesophagus and LES; in Duthie, Gastrointestinal motility in health and disease, MTP Press, Lancaster, 1978, pp. 565-574.
14. Bortolotti M, Labo G. Clinical and manometric effects of nifedipine in patients with esophageal achalasia. *Gastroenterology* 1981; 80: 39-44.
15. Gelfond M, Rozen P, Gilat T. Isosorbide dinitrate and nifedipine treatment of achalasia: a clinical, manometric and radionuclide evaluation. *Gastroenterology* 1982; 83: 963-9.
16. Coccia G, Bortolotti M, Micheti P, Dodero M. Prospective clinical and manometric study comparing pneumatic dilatation and sublingual nifedipine in the treatment of oesophageal achalasia. *Gut* 1991; 32: 604-6.
17. Traube M, Dubovik R, Lange RC, McCallum RW. The role of nifedipine therapy in achalasia: results of a randomized, double-blind placebo-controlled study. *Am J Gastroenterology* 1989; 84: 1259-62.
18. Triadafilopoulos G, Aaronson M, Sackel S, Burakoff R. Medical treatment of esophageal achalasia. Double-blind crossover study with oral nifedipine, verapamil, and placebo. *Dig Dis Sci* 1991; 36: 260-7.
19. Silverstein BD, Kramer CM, Pope CE. Treatment of esophageal motor disorders with a calcium-blocker, diltiazem. *Gastroenterology* 1982; 81: 1181 (abstract).
20. Lorber SM, Shay H. Roentgen studies of esophageal transport in patients with dysphagia due to abnormal motor function. *Gastroenterology* 1955; 28: 697-714.
21. Field C.E. Octyl nitrite in achalasia of the cardia. *Lancet* 1944; 2: 848-51.
22. Douthwaite AJ. Achalasia of cardia. Treatment with nitrites. *Lancet* 1943; 2: 353-4.

23. Gelfond M, Rozen P, Keren S, Gilat T. Effect of nitrates on LOS pressure in achalasia: a potential therapeutic aid. *Gut* 1981; 22: 312-8.
24. Guelrud M, Ramirez M. The effect of transcutaneous nerve stimulation on lower esophageal sphincter pressure in patients with achalasia. *Gastroenterology* 1989; 96: 188.
25. Kaada B. Successful treatment of esophageal dysmotility and Raynaud's phenomenon in systemic sclerosis and achalasia by transcutaneous nerve stimulation. *Scand J Gastroenterol* 1987; 22: 1137.
26. Bennett JR, Hendrix TR. Treatment of achalasia with pneumatic dilatation. *Mod Treat* 1970; 7: 1217.
27. Browne DC, McHardy G. A new instrument for use in esophagospasm. *JAMA* 1992: 1963-4.
28. Csendes A, Strauszer T. Long term clinical, radiological and manometric follow up period of patients with achalasia treated with pneumatic dilatation. *Digestion* 1974; 11: 128-34.
29. Rider JA, Moeller HC, Puletti EJ, Desai DC. Diagnosis and treatment of diffuse esophageal spasm. *Arch Surg* 1969; 99: 435.
30. Vantrappen G, Hellemans J. Treatment of achalasia and related motor disorders. *Gastroenterology* 1980; 79: 144-54.
31. Cox J, Buckton GK, Bennet JR. Balloon dilatation in achalasia: a new dilator. *Gut* 1986; 57: 986.
32. Kadakia SC, Wong RK. Graded pneumatic dilatation using Rigiflex achalasia dilators in patients with primary esophageal achalasia. *Am J Gastroenterol* 1993; 88: 34-8.
33. Lambroza A, Schuman RW. Pneumatic dilatation for achalasia without fluoroscopic guidance: safety and efficacy. *Am J Gastroenterol* 1995; 90: 1226-9.
34. McLean TR, Bombeck CT, Nyhus LM. Endoscopic piggyback pneumatic dilatation in the initial management of patients with achalasia. *Gastrointest Endosc* 1986; 32: 290.
35. Witzel L. Treatment of achalasia with a pneumatic dilator attached to a gastroscope. *Endoscopy* 1981; 13: 176-7.
36. Mearin G, Armengol JR, Chicharro L, Papo M, Balboa A, Malagelada JR. Forceful dilatation under endoscopic control in the treatment of achalasia: a randomized trial of pneumatic *versus* metallic dilator. *Gut* 1994; 35: 1360-2.
37. Tack J, Janssens J, Vantrappen G. Non-surgical treatment of achalasia. *Hepatogastroenterology* 1991; 38: 493-97.
38. Vantrappen G, Hellemans J, Deloof W, Valembois P, Vandenbroucke J. Treatment of achalasia with pneumatic dilatations. *Gut* 1971; 12: 268-75.
39. Reynolds JC, Parkman HP. Achalasia. *Gastroenterol Clin North Am* 1989; 18: 223.
40. Kim CH, Cameron AJ, Hsu JJ, Talley NJ, Trastek VF, Pairolero PC, O'Connor MK, Colwell LJ, Zinsmeister AR. Achalasia: prospective evaluation of relationship between lower esophageal sphincter pressure, esophageal transit, and esophageal diameter and symptoms in response to pneumatic dilatation. *Mayo Clinic Proc* 1993; 68: 1067-73.
41. West RL, Hirsch DP, Bartelsman JFWM, de Borst J, Ferwerda G, Tytgat GNJ, Boeckxstaens GE. Long term results of pneumatic dilatation in achalasia followed for more than 5 years. *The American Journal of Gastroenterology* 2003; 97: 1346-51.
42. Eckardt VF, Aignherr C, Bernhard G. Predictors of outcome in patients with achalasia treated by pneumatic dilatation. *Gastroenterology* 1992; 103: 1732-8.
43. Nair LA, Reynolds JC, Parkman HP, Ouyang A, Strom BL, Rosato EF, Cohen S. Complications during pneumatic dilatation for achalasia or diffuse esophageal spasm. Analysis of risk factors, early clinical characteristics, and outcome. *Dig Dis Sci* 1993; 38: 1893-1904.
44. Pasricha PJ, Ravich WJ, Kalloo AN. Effects of intrasphincteric botulinum toxin on the lower esophageal sphincter in piglets. *Gastroenterology* 1993; 105: 1045-9.
45. Pasricha PJ, Ravich WJ, Hendrix TR, Sostre S, Kalloo AN. Intrasphincteric botulinum toxin for the treatment of achalasia. *New Engl J Med* 1995; 332: 774-8.
46. Pasricha PJ, Rai R, Ravich WJ, Hendrix TR, Kalloo AN. Botulinum toxin for achalasia: long-term outcome and predictors of response. *Gastroenterology* 1996; 110: 1410-5.

47. D'Onofrio V, Annese V, Miletto P, Leandro G, Marasco A, Sodano P, Iaquinto G. Long-term follow-up of patients treated with botulinum toxin. *Diseases of the Esophagus* 2000; 13: 96-101.
48. Muehldorfer SM, Schneider H, Hochberger, J, Martus P, Hagh EG, Ell C. Esophageal achalasia: intrasphincteric injection of botulinum toxin A *versus* balloon dilatation. *Enodsopy* 1999; 31: 517-21.
49. Vaezi MF, Richter JE, Schroeder PL, Birgisson S, Slaugher RL, Koehler RE, Baker ME. Botulinum toxin *versus* pneumatic dilatation in the treatment of achalasia: a randomised trial. *Gut* 1999; 44: 231-9.
50. Black J, Vorbach AN, Collis JL. Results of Heller's operation for achalasia of the esophagus. The importance of hiatal repair. *Br J Surg* 1976; 63; 949-53.
51. Csendes A, Larrain A, Strauszer T, Ayala M. Long term clinical, radiological and manometric follow up period of patients with achalasia of the esophagus treated with esophagomyotomy. *Digestion* 1975; 13; 141-5.
52. Effler DB, Loop FL, Groves LK, Favaloro AG. Primary surgical treatment for esophageal achalasia. *Surg Gynecol Obstet* 1971; 132; 1057-63.
53. Ellis FH, Gibb SP, Grozier RE. Esophagomyotomy for achalasia of the esophagus. *Ann Surg* 1980; 192: 157-61.
54. Jara FM, Toledo-Pereyra LH, Lewis JW, Magilligan DJ. Long-term results of esophagomyotomy for achalasia of esophagus. *Arch Surg* 1979; 114: 935-6.
55. Menguy R. Management of achalasia by transabdominal cardiomyotomy and funduplication. *Surg Gynecol Obstet* 1971; 133; 482-4.
56. Menzies-Gow N, Gummer JWP, Edwards DAW. Results of Heller's operation for achalasia of the cardia. *Br J Surg* 1978; 65; 483-5.
57. Rees JR, Thorbjarnarson B, Barnes WH. Achalasia: results of operations in 84 patients. *Ann Surg* 1970; 171: 195-201.
58. Wingfield MV, Karwowski A. The treatment of achalasia by cardiomyotomy. *Br J Surg* 1972; 59: 281-4.
59. Vantrappen G, Janssens J. To dilate or to operate? That is the question. *Gut* 1983; 24: 1013.
60. Parkman HP, Reynolds JC, Ouyang A, Rosato EF, Eisenberg JM, Cohen S. Pneumatic dilatation or esophagomyotomy treatment for idiopathic achalasia: clinical outcomes and cost analysis. *Dig Dis Sci* 1993; 38: 75-85.
61. Csendes A, Velasco N, Braghetto I, Henriquez A. A prospective randomized study comparing forceful dilatation and oesophagomyotomy in patients with achalasia of the oesophagus. *Gastroenterology* 1981; 80: 789-95.
62. Csendes A, Braghetto I, Henriquez A, Cortes A. Late results of a prospective randomised study comparing forceful dilatation and oesophagomyotomy in patients with achalasia. *Gut* 1989; 30: 299-304.
63. Okike N, Spencer Payne W, Neufeld DM, Bernatz PE, Pairolero PC, Sanderson DR. Oesophagomyotomy *versus* forceful dilatation for achalasia of the oesophagus: results in 899 patients. *Ann Thorac Surg* 1979; 28: 119-25.

Long-term results and outcome of minimally invasive surgical treatment of GERD

Bernard Dallemagne

Department of Digestive Surgery, CHC-Les Cliniques Saint-Joseph, Liege, Belgium

Since our initial report of the laparoscopic approach of Nissen fundoplication in 1991 [1], there has been a large acceptance of the technique by the surgical community. Hundreds of papers have been published, reactivating the long debate about the need for surgical therapy of gastroesophageal reflux disease (GERD) and the best type of operation.

Short-term results of laparoscopic antireflux surgery are equivalent to those of open approach but information on longer-term outcome is required to confirm its durability [2-5]. During this period, alarming reports have been published concerning the usefulness of the operation. The long-term follow-up of a randomized trial demonstrates that more than 60% of operated patients are back to antacid medications [6].

This report has to be confronted to the published long-term results of laparoscopic fundoplication and to our own experience.

Methods

A review of the current available literature on laparoscopic fundoplication has been made trough a Pubmed search with mesh requirements focused on long-term results, *i.e.* papers published after year 2000. In this series, papers reporting on follow-up longer than five years were kept for analysis.

The second step was to analyze the long-term data of a cohort of 100 consecutive patients operated in 1993, by a single surgeon, in our hospital. The real follow-up duration was over ten years.

Results

Review of the literature

There were six relevant publications addressing outcome of at least five years after laparoscopic fundoplication [7-12] *(table I)*.

Table I. Relevant publications on long term follow-up after laparoscopic fundoplication

Author	N	FUP	Good-excellent	Re-op.	ppi
Bammer 2001 [8]	171	Mean: 6.4 years	96%	3%	14%
Booth 2002 [9]	48	Median: 6 years	93%	6%	14%
Lafullarde 2002 [11]	176	Mean: 6 years	90%	13%	
Kamoltz 2002 [10]	169	> 5 years	97.9%	5.7%	nc
Anvari 2002 [7]	181	> 5 years	88%	4%	12%
Nilsson 2004 [12]	22	> 5 years	98%	6%	4.5%

Re-op = re operation rate (%); ppi: % of patients using Proton Pump Inhibitors.

Control of reflux symptoms is obtained in 88% to 98% of patients. Most of the follow-up results are based on a subjective evaluation of symptoms and/or indexes of quality of life. Reoperation rate is around 5-6%, except for one report. Causes of redo surgery are paraesophageal herniation, dysphagia and recurrence. Four to fourteen percent of patients are back to antacid therapy, some of them for non-GERD symptoms.

Personal series

In 1993, 165 patients underwent laparoscopic Nissen or Toupet (partial posterior) fundoplication in our department. From this surgical series, 100 consecutive patients operated by a single surgeon were extracted. There were 38 women and 62 men. The median age of the patients was 52 (range 10-78 years).

All patients underwent upper gastrointestinal endoscopy. Oesophagitis was scored using the classification of Savary and Miller. Twelve patients had grade 1 esophagitis, 67 grade 2, 6 grade 3, 15 had Barrett's esophagus. Twenty-four hour ambulatory pH monitoring was performed before operation in 60 patients. Abnormal deMeester's score was demonstrated in 57 patients.

All but one (10 years old) patients underwent standard esophageal manometry. Nineteen patients had residual pressure (> 6 mmHg) in the lower esophageal sphincter (LES); eighty patients presented with LES pressure lower than 6 mmHg, and normal motility (n = 54), or impaired esophageal peristalsis (n = 26). All patients underwent upper GI series before operation. A hiatus hernia was demonstrated in 71 patients, reducible in upright position in 81% of them.

Operative techniques

Two types of fundoplication were performed in this series.

Laparoscopic Nissen fundoplication was performed in 68 patients by fashioning a floppy 360° wrap with routine division of the short gastric vessels. A < 2 cm wrap was created with non absorbable sutures. The wrap was not anchored to the crura.

Laparoscopic partial posterior fundoplication was performed in 32 patients by fashioning a 270° posterior wrap with routine division of the short gastric vessels. The 4 cm wrap was anchored to the right and left crura.

Choice between these two fundoplications was based on the results of the esophageal manometry, and per-operative anatomical factors (size of the gastric fundus).

Postoperative assessment

This series of 100 patients was analyzed after a follow-up period of time of five years (unpublished data): patient symptom information was obtained using a standardized symptom questionnaire. Patients were asked to grade the following symptoms on a four-point scale (0, absent; 1, mild; 2, moderate; 3, severe): heartburn, regurgitation, dysphagia, chest pain, nausea, belching, abdominal distension, flatulence,) and medication taken. Images of the fundoplication were obtained with barium swallow. Correlation between X rays and symptoms were made.

Ten years after surgery, this series of patient was reanalyzed using the same symptom questionnaire and a quality of life questionnaire, the Gastrointestinal Quality of Life (GIQLI) that was developed by Eyspach *et al.* [13]. The questionnaire contains up to 36 items, scored on a five point Likert scale (range 0-144, higher score =better quality of life) The scores of each item are used to calculate a score between 0 and 4 for each of the five subdimensions: gastrointestinal (GI) symptoms, emotional status, physical functions, social functions, and stress by medical treatment. Higher scores reflect a better quality of life. The mean GIQLI of healthy controls is 122.6 ± 8.5 points.

Long-term follow-up was performed in all patients by postal survey and by hospital visit, if accepted by the patient.

Results

There was no death related to surgery. There was no conversion to open procedure.

The post-fundoplication history of this group of patient is schematized in *table II*.

Sixty of the 87 available patients at ten years responded to the two questionnaires.

Table II. Outcome of 100 patients after laparoscopic fundoplication performed in 1993

1993		1998		2004
100 patients	2 reoperations	95 patients	2 reoperations	87 patients
68 Nissen fundoplications	1 gastrectomy	Symptom questionnaire	1 obesity surgery	Symptom questionnaire
32 Toupet fundoplications	2 deaths	Barium swallow	5 deaths	GIQLI
		Response: 86 patients (90.5%)		Response: 64 patients (73.5%)

Four patients responded only to the ten years questionnaire. Twenty-two patients responded only to the first mailing.

When cumulating the two questionnaires, there are only three patients lost for any follow-up.

• **At five years follow-up**, there were two patients who required revisional surgery: one for persisting dysphagia, one for recurrent symptoms. Overall 93% of patients were free from significant reflux symptoms, *i.e.* scores for heartburn, regurgitations and retrosternal pain were one or less (Nissen: 95.6%; Toupet: 85.6%).

Antacid therapy was used in eleven patients (12.7%: six Toupet's patient (21%) and five Nissen's patient (8%).

There were no statistical differences in term of side effects (dysphagia, flatulence, abdominal distension).

When analyzing the relationship between reflux symptoms and barium swallow *(table III)* one can see that the incidence of wrap migration was significantly higher in the Toupet's group, leading to recurrent symptoms in two patients.

• **From 5 years to 10 years follow-up**, two patients from the Toupet's group required reoperation for recurrence demonstrated at five years follow-up.

Table III. Impact of anatomical wrap position on the outcome (heartburn) of partial and total fundoplication

Heartburn (score)	Toupet	Nissen
None (0)	3/13 intrathoracic migration	32/32 valve well positionned
Occasional (1)	2/4 intrathoracic migration	6/6 valve well positionned
Therapy (2)	2/2 intrathoracic migration	0
Severe (3)	0	0

- **At 10 years follow-up**, 87 patients were available for study. Sixty-four patients returned the postal questionnaire (response rate: 73.5%). Overall 92% of patients were free from significant reflux symptoms. Control of reflux was obtained in 93% after Nissen and 88% of patients after Toupet fundoplication.

Eight patients used PPIs: five of them were already taking this medication at five years.

The mean GIQLI score for the whole group was 113.5 (95%CI 107-119); mean score for Nissen group was 115.3 and 108.7 for Toupet group (no significant). It has to be compared to the mean GIQLI score in the normal population (122.6) and to our preoperative score, under medical therapy (mean score 94).

- **News from the patients who respond only to the first questionnaire (20 patients)**

One patient has a breast cancer; one patient has a lung cancer. We have no news from 13 patients. Five patients had contact with our institution during the past year and were free of recurrent symptoms.

In summary, from this initial series of 100 patients, seven patients died from unrelated disease. Four patients (4%) underwent reoperation, one for dysphagia, and three for recurrent reflux.

Discussion

Antireflux surgery has an established place in the treatment of GERD. The goal of the operation is resolution of all symptoms of GERD with negligible side effects and no further need for medical therapy.

A number of long-term studies of open fundoplications have been published. Reported success rates vary between 76% in one 20-year follow-up study and 91% in an extrapolated actuarial analysis [14-17]. Others have described return of reflux esophagitis in more than 50% of cases within six years.

Spechler *et al.* reported a 62% rate of use of antireflux medications after surgical fundoplication in a randomized controlled trial of open fundoplication *vs* medical [18]. Mean duration of follow-up was 10.6 years for medical patients and 9.1 years for surgical patients. However, 86% of surgical patients were satisfied with the results of the operation. Interestingly, there were no significant differences between medical and surgical groups in the frequency of increased abdominal fullness, inability to belch, inability to vomit and increased abdominal girth.

There have been major changes during the past decade. Since its introduction in 1991, the laparoscopic technique has replaced open antireflux operation as the method of choice. Less surgical trauma, reduced pain, shorter hospital stay and sick leave and cosmetically more acceptable scars are some of the proposed advantages.

It is assumed that laparoscopic surgery will give at least equal results to open procedures. Many studies report excellent short-term results after laparoscopic antireflux surgery [19-24]. Some randomized control trials published similar short-term results for both techniques.

However some reports have emphasized on the large incidence of early post-laparoscopic complications and reoperation rates [25, 26]. The long learning curve of the laparoscopic technique has been identified as a confounding factor [27, 28]. Reports of the long-term results of this appealing technique are few in number. Good to excellent results after follow-up longer than five years are obtained in approximately 90% of patients, taking in consideration a reoperation rates that vary between 4 and 13%.

Our analysis of patients at 5 and more than 10-year follow-up revealed a rate of control of reflux symptoms in over 90% of patients. Twelve percent of patients are taking antacid medications, some of them without obvious recurrent reflux symptoms, in the context of Barrett's esophagus or gastric diseases. This is far away from some published results of 60% of patients back on medication after surgery.

Analysis of paired data at 5 year and 10-year follow-up revealed stabilization of the results. Reoperation was necessary in four patients within the first five years.

Concerning the anatomical results of the fundoplications, barium swallow studies performed five years after operation demonstrate a well-shaped and positioned valve in all patients after Nissen fundoplication and an intrathoracic migration of a partial posterior fundoplication in 7/19 patients. Of these, only two patients required therapy for recurrent symptoms. One of them underwent remedial surgery few months after the study. Three of these patients are free of symptoms at ten years. The results of this barium swallow study differ from some reports that demonstrate anatomical failure rate of the fundoplication in up to 55% of patients [29].

Compared to some long-term series, we did not experience the same incidence of typical laparoscopic early postoperative complication, such as paraesophageal herniation. This is probably related to the surgical technique, in which we were used to perform a systematic crural repair. One patient with a Barrett's esophagus was reoperated for persisting dysphagia. Conversion to partial posterior did not solve the problem, which was related to primary esophageal motility disorders. Our zero rate of disturbing postoperative dysphagia is probably related to the construction of a very floppy valve, thanks to a systematic fundic mobilization. This technical point has however not been confirmed by some randomized trials [22, 30, 31]. Technical differences in the quality of this gastric mobilization might explain our excellent results. Main reported side effects are related to abdominal distension and flatulence, mainly at the end of the day. More than forty percent of patients report this complain, with a rate that is stable between five and ten years. Unfortunately, in our study, these symptoms were not scored preoperatively and cannot be evaluated properly.

At long-term, it appears that laparoscopic fundoplication reproduces the results of open fundoplication as demonstrated in some studies. After open operations, there are statistically more complains about scars. The other parameters seem to be equivalent: control of symptoms, side effects [12]. But we have to bear in mind that these results are obtained at the price of a reduced operative mortality and morbidity rate, shorter hospital stay and sick leave, lower incidence of incisional complications. There is also a substantial reduction in the number of "accidental" splenectomies, as they were reported in the open experience (0-8%) [32-34]. In total, if the results of other long-term studies confirm the results obtained in well trained and dedicated surgical centers, laparoscopic fundoplication might become the gold standard of treatment of gastro-esophageal reflux disease in appropriately investigated and selected patients.

References

1. Dallemagne B, Weerts JM, Jehaes C, Markiewicz S, Lombard R. Laparoscopic Nissen fundoplication: preliminary report. *Surg Laparosc Endosc* 1991; 1: 138-43.
2. Heikkinen TJ, Haukipuro K, Bringman S, Ramel S, Sorasto A, Hulkko A. Comparison of laparoscopic and open Nissen fundoplication 2 years after operation. A prospective randomized trial. *Surg Endosc* 2000; 14: 1019-23.
3. Laine S, Rantala A, Gullichsen R, Ovaska J. Laparoscopic *vs* conventional Nissen fundoplication. A prospective randomized study. *Surg Endosc* 1997; 11: 441-4.
4. Majeed AW, Johnson AG. Randomized clinical trial of laparoscopic *versus* open fundoplication: blind evaluation of recovery and discharge period. *Br J Surg* 2000; 87: 1735.
5. Nilsson G, Larsson S, Johnsson F. Randomized clinical trial of laparoscopic *versus* open fundoplication: blind evaluation of recovery and discharge period. *Br J Surg* 2000; 87: 873-8.
6. Spechler SJ, Lee E, Ahnen D, Goyal RK, Hirano I, Ramirez F, Raufman JP, Sampliner R, Schnell T, Sontag S, Vlahcevic ZR, Young R, Williford W. Long-term outcome of medical and surgical therapies for gastroesophageal reflux disease: follow-up of a randomized controlled trial. *JAMA* 2001; 285: 2331-8.
7. Anvari M, Allen C. Five-year comprehensive outcomes evaluation in 181 patients after laparoscopic Nissen fundoplication. *J Am Coll Surg* 2003; 196: 51-7.
8. Bammer T, Hinder RA, Klaus A, Klingler PJ. Five- to eight-year outcome of the first laparoscopic Nissen fundoplications. *J Gastrointest Surg* 2001; 5: 42-8.
9. Booth MI, Jones L, Stratford J, Dehn TC. Results of laparoscopic Nissen fundoplication at 2-8 years after surgery. *Br J Surg* 2002; 89: 476-81.
10. Kamolz T, Granderath FA, Bammer T, Wykypiel H, Jr., Pointner R, Floppy. Nissen *vs* Toupet laparoscopic fundoplication: quality of life assessment in a 5-year follow-up (part 2). *Endoscopy* 2002; 34: 917-22.
11. Lafullarde T, Watson DI, Jamieson GG, Myers JC, Game PA, Devitt PG. Laparoscopic Nissen fundoplication: five-year results and beyond. *Arch Surg* 2001; 136: 180-4.
12. Nilsson G, Wenner J, Larsson S, Johnsson F. Randomized clinical trial of laparoscopic *versus* open fundoplication for gastro-oesophageal reflux. *Br J Surg* 2004; 91: 552-9.
13. Eypasch E, Williams JI, Wood-Dauphinee S, Ure BM, Schmulling C, Neugebauer E, Troidl H. Gastrointestinal Quality of Life Index: development, validation and application of a new instrument. *Br J Surg* 1995; 82: 216-22.
14. DeMeester TR, Bonavina L, Albertucci M. Nissen fundoplication for gastroesophageal reflux disease. Evaluation of primary repair in 100 consecutive patients. *Ann Surg* 1986; 204: 9-20.
15. Grande L, Toledo-Pimentel V, Manterola C, Lacima G, Ros E, Garcia-Valdecasas JC, Fuster J, Visa J, Pera C. Value of Nissen fundoplication in patients with gastro-oesophageal reflux judged by long-term symptom control. *Br J Surg* 1994; 81: 548-50.

16. Lundell L, Miettinen P, Myrvold HE, Pedersen SA, Liedman B, Hatlebakk JG, Julkonen R, Levander K, Carlsson J, Lamm M, Wiklund I. Continued (5-year) followup of a randomized clinical study comparing antireflux surgery and omeprazole in gastroesophageal reflux disease. *J Am Coll Surg* 2001; 192: 172-9.
17. Luostarinen M, Isolauri J, Laitinen J, Koskinen M, Keyrilainen O, Markkula H, Lehtinen E, Uusitalo A. Fate of Nissen fundoplication after 20 years. A clinical, endoscopical, and functional analysis. *Gut* 1993; 34: 1015-20.
18. Spechler SJ, Lee E, Ahnen D, Goyal RK, Hirano I, Ramirez F, Raufman JP, Sampliner R, Schnell T, Sontag S, Vlahcevic ZR, Young R, Williford W. Long-term outcome of medical and surgical therapies for gastroesophageal reflux disease: follow-up of a randomized controlled trial. *JAMA* 2001; 285: 2331-8.
19. Hinder RA, Filipi CJ, Wetscher G, Neary P, DeMeester TR, Perdikis G. Laparoscopic Nissen fundoplication is an effective treatment for gastroesophageal reflux disease. *Ann Surg* 1994; 220: 472-81.
20. Hunter JG, Trus TL, Branum GD, Waring JP, Wood WC. A physiologic approach to laparoscopic fundoplication for gastroesophageal reflux disease. *Ann Surg* 1996; 223: 673-85.
21. Lundell L. Anti-reflux surgery in the laparoscopic era. *Baillieres Best Pract Res Clin Gastroenterol* 2000; 14: 793-810.
22. O'Boyle CJ, Watson DI, Jamieson GG, Myers JC, Game PA, Devitt PG. Division of short gastric vessels at laparoscopic nissen fundoplication: a prospective double-blind randomized trial with 5-year follow-up. *Ann Surg* 2002; 235: 165-70.
23. Patti MG, Feo CV, De Pinto M, Arcerito M, Tong J, Gantert W, Tyrrell D, Way LW. Results of laparoscopic antireflux surgery for dysphagia and gastroesophageal reflux disease. *Am J Surg* 1998; 176: 564-8.
24. Peters JH, DeMeester TR, Crookes P, Oberg S, de Vos SM, Hagen JA, Bremner CG. The treatment of gastroesophageal reflux disease with laparoscopic Nissen fundoplication: prospective evaluation of 100 patients with typical symptoms. *Ann Surg* 1998; 228: 40-50.
25. Dallemagne B, Weerts JM, Jehaes C, Markiewicz S. Causes of failures of laparoscopic antireflux operations. *Surg Endosc* 1996; 10: 305-10.
26. Watson DI, Jamieson GG, Devitt PG, Mitchell PC, Game PA. Paraoesophageal hiatus hernia: an important complication of laparoscopic Nissen fundoplication. *Br J Surg* 1995; 82: 521-3.
27. Voitk A, Joffe J, Alvarez C, Rosenthal G. Factors contributing to laparoscopic failure during the learning curve for laparoscopic Nissen fundoplication in a community hospital. *J Laparoendosc Adv Surg Tech A* 1999; 9: 243-8.
28. Watson DI, Jamieson GG, Baigrie RJ, Mathew G, Devitt PG, Game PA, Britten-Jones R. Laparoscopic surgery for gastro-oesophageal reflux: beyond the learning curve. *Br J Surg* 1996; 83: 1284-7.
29. Donkervoort SC, Bais JE, Rijnhart-de Jong H, Gooszen HG. Impact of anatomical wrap position on the outcome of Nissen fundoplication. *Br J Surg* 2003; 90: 854-9.
30. Chrysos E, Tzortzinis A, Tsiaoussis J, Athanasakis H, Vasssilakis J, Xynos E. Prospective randomized trial comparing Nissen to Nissen-Rossetti technique for laparoscopic fundoplication. *Am J Surg* 2001; 182: 215-21.
31. Luostarinen ME, Isolauri JO. Randomized trial to study the effect of fundic mobilization on long-term results of Nissen fundoplication. *Br J Surg* 1999; 86: 614-8.
32. Stein HJ, Feussner H, Siewert JR. Antireflux surgery: a current comparison of open and laparoscopic approaches. *Hepatogastroenterology* 1998; 45: 1328-37.
33. Urschel JD. Complications of antireflux surgery. *Am J Surg* 1993; 166: 68-70.
34. Viljakka MT, Luostarinen ME, Isolauri JO. Complications of open and laparoscopic antireflux surgery: 32-year audit at a teaching hospital. *J Am Coll Surg* 1997; 185: 446-50.
35. Booth MI, Jones L, Stratford J, Dehn TC. Results of laparoscopic Nissen fundoplication at 2-8 years after surgery. *Br J Surg* 2002; 89: 476-81.

Management of bleeding esophageal varices: endoscopy or TIPS?

Henk R. van Buuren

Department of Gastroenterology & Hepatology, Erasmus Medical Centre Rotterdam, Rotterdam, The Netherlands

Bleeding from esophago-gastric varices remains a catastrophic medical event, with reported mortality rates ranging from 10-40%. The main predictor for outcome is liver function. Other reported prognostic factors include portal pressure, the presence of infection and active bleeding at the initial endoscopy.

A recent meta-analysis suggests that the combination of endoscopic treatment and vasoactive drugs (*e.g.* terlipressin, somatostatin, octreotide) [1] is superior to endoscopic treatment alone in patients with acute variceal bleeding. Prophylactic administration of antibiotics in patients with cirrhosis and gastrointestinal haemorrhage has been shown to significantly reduce the incidence of infections and to improve survival [2]. Consequently, many centres have now adopted a policy of standard triple therapy, consisting of endoscopic treatment, vaso-active drugs and antibiotics. This approach has been advocated during the last international Baveno consensus meeting on portal hypertension [3].

After the acute bleeding episode the two main treatment options are non-selective β-blockers (propranolol or nadolol) and endoscopic treatment [3].

The Transjugular Intrahepatic Portosystemic Shunt procedure (TIPS) was introduced into clinical practice in 1988 and is now the principal modality to treat those patients in whom other therapies, either to control acute bleeding or to prevent recurrent bleeding, fail [3]. Although controlled comparative studies have not been performed, it is generally accepted that TIPS is a valuable "salvage" treatment in these situations. We will focus here on the question whether TIPS should also be considered as a first-line treatment modality in variceal bleeding.

Endoscopic therapy vs TIPS

Fourteen comparative trials of TIPS *versus* endoscopic treatment have been reported, either as full reports [4-15], in abstract form [16] or as part of a thesis [17]. In three studies endoscopic therapy was combined with propranolol [5, 6, 15] *(table I)*. In none of these trials coated stents for TIPS were used. All trials except two [7, 14] found TIPS to be superior in the prevention of variceal rebleeding. However, in only one trial this was associated with improved overall survival [11]. Nearly all studies found the incidence of hepatic encephalopathy to be higher in patients treated with TIPS. These findings have been confirmed by meta-analyses [18-20].

Table I. Randomized controlled trials of TIPS *versus* endoscopic treatment: trial characteristics

Trial	Year	No. of patients (TIPS/endoscopic)	Type of endoscopic treatment	Follow-up (months)
GEAIH [16]	1995	32/33	Sclerotherapy	12 (mean)
Cabrera [4]	1996	31/32	Sclerotherapy	15 (mean)
Rössle [5]	1997	61/65	Sclerotherapy, banding ligation, propranolol	14 (median)
Sauer [6]	1997	42/41	Sclerotherapy + propranolol	18 (median)
Sanyal [7]	1997	41/39	Sclerotherapy	32 (median)
Cello [8]	1997	24/25	Sclerotherapy	19 (mean)
Jalan [9]	1997	31/27	Band ligation	16 (mean)
Merli [10]	1998	38/43	Sclerotherapy	18 (mean)
Garcia-Villareal [11]	1999	22/24	Sclerotherapy	20 (mean)
Pomier-Layrargues [12]	2001	41/39	Band ligation	20 (mean)
Narahara [13]	2001	38/40	Sclerotherapy	36 (mean)
Gulberg [14]	2002	28/26	Band ligation	24 (mean)
Sauer [15]	2002	43/42	Band ligation + propranolol	46 (mean)
Van Buuren [17]	2002	19/18	Band ligation	21 (mean)

Why does TIPS, while being more effective in preventing rebleeding, not reduce mortality?

The first question is whether TIPS decreases the mortality associated with recurrent variceal bleeding. In a meta-analysis of Luca *et al.* [19] this effect was not significant. In a meta-analysis of 10 trials [4-8, 10-12, 17, 19] we found that 9/326 (3%) patients died of variceal bleeding after TIPS and 30/328 (9%) treated endoscopically. This difference was statistically significant (Mantel-Haenszel method; p = 0.01; odds ratio 3.4; 95% CI 1-6-7.4).

The next question is why TIPS, despite being more effective in terms of prevention of (mortality due to) rebleeding, fails to improve overall survival. One factor involved may be that in all studies patients assigned to endoscopic therapy were allowed to crossover to shunt implantation when they failed therapy. In the reported trials this "rescue by TIPS" occurred in 4-30% of patients assigned to endoscopic treatment, and it is likely that these patients had a high mortality risk at the time of cross-over. Therefore, this cross-over may have obscured treatment effects of TIPS, although it has been argued that this may not be factor of decisive importance [20]. Also, TIPS creation may be associated with more (fatal) procedure related complications. Although fatal complications after TIPS, including hemoperitoneum [6, 7, 12] and perforation of the portal vein [9], have been reported, further evaluation of the trial data shows no clear differences between treatment groups. Another possibility is that TIPS adversely affects liver function, resulting in higher mortality from liver failure. However, the combined data of the previously mentioned trials [4-8, 10-12, 17, 19] indicate that 26/326 (11%) shunted patients died of liver failure compared to 27/328 endoscopically treated patients (odds ratio 0.7; 95% CI 0.4-1,3). Fatal infections were reported more frequently after TIPS (TIPS 4,8%, endoscopic therapy 2,7%), but this difference is not significant. No other clear differences between both treatment options are apparent with respect to other causes of death. For the time being, it is difficult to find a satisfactory explanation for the unaltered mortality risk after TIPS. Possible factors involved are the treatment crossover phenomenon and the presence of a type II statistical error.

Costs of TIPS in comparison with endoscopic treatment

Data on the relative costs of TIPS and endoscopic therapy are scarce and literature data do not seem to allow firm conclusions [18]. Several studies found no difference with respect to the re-admission rate to hospital [7, 11, 12] or costs [8]. However, this has not been a uniform finding and both higher [21] and lower [9] costs associated with TIPS have been reported.

Current consensus: TIPS or endoscopic therapy?

TIPS is clearly superior to endoscopic therapy in the prevention of variceal rebleeding. However, given the absence of a survival benefit, the increased risk for encephalopathy and the absence of a clearly documented advantage with respect to costs, the current recommendation is not to use TIPS as the first line therapy in variceal bleeding [3].

Gastric variceal bleeding

There are no solid data indicating the superiority of one over other treatment option in gastric variceal bleeding. Several centers have reported on TIPS as an effective treatment when endoscopic and other therapies fail [22, 23]. For the time being, TIPS is a reasonable treatment option, particularly in patients with major bleeding preventing adequate visualisation and endoscopic therapy, recurrent bleeding after previous endoscopic treatment *(figure 1)* or with other complications such as refractory ascites. Obviously data derived from controlled investigations are urgently needed. Especially, TIPS should be compared with endoscopic glue injection.

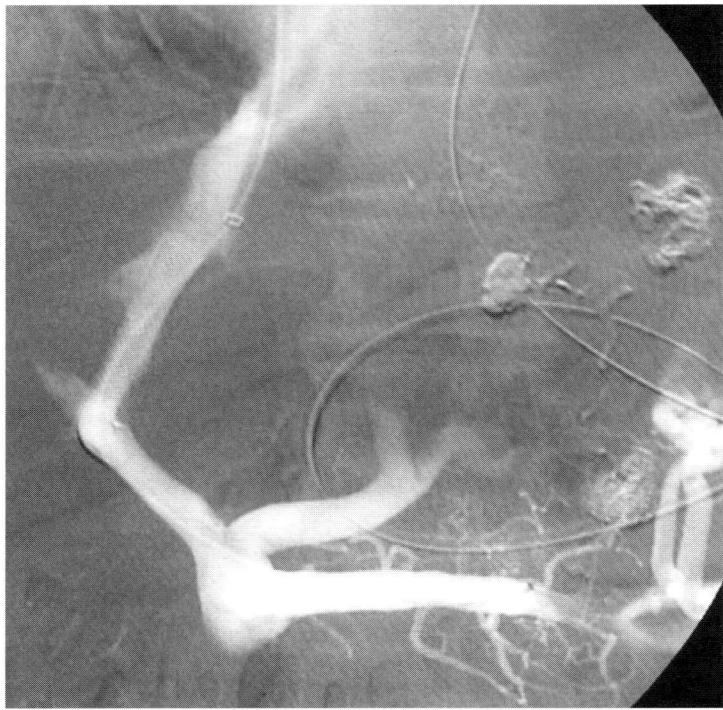

Figure 1. Portography after TIPS creation in a patient with recurrent bleeding from large gastric varices. Histoacryl®-Lipiodol® accumulations are visible after (unsuccessful) endoscopic injection treatment of the gastric varices as well as an enlarged coronary vein and large splenic-gastric collaterals.

Ectopic variceal bleeding

Bleeding from varices outside the gastro-esophageal junction area is rare. Bleeding from rectal, duodenal, enterostomal, peritoneal and other types of ectopic varices can be managed with local therapies including injection therapy, band ligation, local sutures or reinsertion of stomas but, at least in our experience, such therapies frequently fail. TIPS has been reported to be effective in a number of cases [24-29]. No controlled studies in this area have been reported.

Prophylactic TIPS?

Considering the potential adverse effect on liver function, risk for encephalopathy and the availability of less invasive alternatives such as propranolol and band ligation, TIPS does not seem indicated for the primary prophylaxis of variceal bleeding. Nevertheless, in a small number of patients with portal hypertension scheduled for abdominal surgery [30], renal transplantation [31] or endoscopic mucosal resection [32], TIPS implantation prior to the procedure has been used in an attempt to prevent complications and lower surgical morbidity. Clearly, such policy is not supported by results of controlled trials. Prophylactic TIPS in surgical patients should be considered cautiously, taking all individual and surgical aspects into consideration.

The future – new trials with new stents?

Several non-controlled series [33-35] and one controlled trial [36] unequivocally show that the incidence of shunt dysfunction is significantly lower when stents covered with polytetrafluoroethylene (e-PTFE) are used for TIPS. In the controlled trial by Bureau *et al.* [36] shunt dysfunction after insertion of a e-PTFE coated stent occurred in 5/39 patients compared to 18/41 patients treated with conventional, non-coated stents ($p < 0.001$). For the group treated with TIPS for digestive bleeding, recurrent haemorrhage was noted in 2/19 patients receiving coated stents compared to 4/29 receiving conventional stents. Ascites recurred in 1/20 patients with ascites receiving coated stents and in 8/12 patients with conventional stents. Surprisingly, the risk for encephalopathy was lower in the group receiving a coated stent ($p = 0.058$). The authors speculate that this might be attributable to the lower number of clinical relapses and the subsequent lower requirement of hospitalisations, invasive procedures and reintervention. Other potential factors involved may be the lower need of diuretic treatment and improved nutritional status of particularly those patients with refractory patients. Although the 1- and 2 year probability of survival was higher in the group treated with coated stents, this difference was not statistically significant.

Given these data it seems appropriate to reconsider the role of TIPS in the management of patients with variceal bleeding. New trials could be initiated to compare TIPS (with implantation of coated stents) with the best endoscopic treatment option, variceal band ligation. A key aspect would be to assess the risk for encephalopathy, particularly the risk for chronic, invalidating and difficult to treat encephalopathy. After all, portosystemic shunting is handling a double-edged sword, requiring great skills to maintain the delicate balance between adequate portal decompression and serious adverse effects (encephalopathy, liver failure).

References

1. Banares R, Albillos A, Rincon D, Alonso S, Gonzalez M, Ruiz-del-Arbol L, et al. Endoscopic treatment *versus* endoscopic plus pharmacologic treatment for acute variceal bleeding: a meta-analysis. *Hepatology* 2002; 35: 609-15.
2. Bernard B, Grange JD, Khac EN, Amiot X, Opolon P, Poynard T. Antibiotic prophylaxis for the prevention of bacterial infections in cirrhotic patients with gastrointestinal bleeding: a meta-analysis. *Hepatology* 1999; 29: 1655-61.
3. De Franchis R. Updating consensus in portal hypertension: report of the Baveno III Consensus Workshop on definitions, methodology and therapeutic strategies in portal hypertension. *J Hepatol* 2000; 33: 846-52.
4. Cabrera J, Maynar M, Granados R, Gorriz E, Reyes R, Pulido-Duque JM, et al. Transjugular intrahepatic portosystemic shunt *versus* sclerotherapy in the elective treatment of variceal hemorrhage. *Gastroenterology* 1996; 110: 832-9.
5. Rossle M, Deibert P, Haag K, Ochs A, Olschewski M, Siegerstetter V, et al. Randomised trial of transjugular-intrahepatic-portosystemic shunt *versus* endoscopy plus propranolol for prevention of variceal rebleeding. *Lancet* 1997; 349: 1043-9.
6. Sauer P, Theilmann L, Stremmel W, Benz C, Richter GM, Stiehl A. Transjugular intrahepatic portosystemic stent shunt *versus* sclerotherapy plus propranolol for variceal rebleeding. *Gastroenterology* 1997; 113: 1623-31.
7. Sanyal AJ, Freedman AM, Luketic VA, Purdum PP, 3rd, Shiffman ML, Cole PE, et al. Transjugular intrahepatic portosystemic shunts compared with endoscopic sclerotherapy for the prevention of recurrent variceal hemorrhage. A randomized, controlled trial. *Ann Intern Med* 1997; 126: 849-57.
8. Cello JP, Ring EJ, Olcott EW, Koch J, Gordon R, Sandhu J, et al. Endoscopic sclerotherapy compared with percutaneous transjugular intrahepatic portosystemic shunt after initial sclerotherapy in patients with acute variceal hemorrhage. A randomized, controlled trial. *Ann Intern Med* 1997; 126: 858-65.
9. Jalan R, Forrest EH, Stanley AJ, Redhead DN, Forbes J, Dillon JF, et al. A randomized trial comparing transjugular intrahepatic portosystemic stent-shunt with variceal band ligation in the prevention of rebleeding from esophageal varices. *Hepatology* 1997; 26: 1115-22.
10. Merli M, Salerno F, Riggio O, de Franchis R, Fiaccadori F, Meddi P, et al. Transjugular intrahepatic portosystemic shunt *versus* endoscopic sclerotherapy for the prevention of variceal bleeding in cirrhosis: a randomized multicenter trial. Gruppo Italiano Studio TIPS (GIST). *Hepatology* 1998; 27: 48-53.
11. Garcia-Villarreal L, Martinez-Lagares F, Sierra A, Guevara C, Marrero JM, Jimenez E, et al. Transjugular intrahepatic portosystemic shunt *versus* endoscopic sclerotherapy for the prevention of variceal rebleeding after recent variceal hemorrhage. *Hepatology* 1999; 29: 27-32.
12. Pomier-Layrargues G, Villeneuve JP, Deschenes M, Bui B, Perreault P, Fenyves D, et al. Transjugular intrahepatic portosystemic shunt (TIPS) *versus* endoscopic variceal ligation in the prevention of variceal rebleeding in patients with cirrhosis: a randomised trial. *Gut* 2001; 48: 390-6.
13. Narahara Y, Kanazawa H, Kawamata H, Tada N, Saitoh H, Matsuzaka S, et al. A randomized clinical trial comparing transjugular intrahepatic portosystemic shunt with endoscopic sclerotherapy in the long-term management of patients with cirrhosis after recent variceal hemorrhage. *Hepatol Res* 2001; 21: 189-98.
14. Gulberg V, Schepke M, Geigenberger G, Holl J, Brensing KA, Waggershauser T, et al. Transjugular intrahepatic portosystemic shunting is not superior to endoscopic variceal band ligation for prevention of variceal rebleeding in cirrhotic patients: a randomized, controlled trial. *Scand J Gastroenterol* 2002; 37: 338-43.
15. Sauer P, Hansmann J, Richter GM, Stremmel W, Stiehl A. Endoscopic variceal ligation plus propranolol *vs* transjugular intrahepatic portosystemic stent shunt: a long-term randomized trial. *Endoscopy* 2002; 34: 690-7.

16. Groupe d'Etude des Anastomoses Intra-Hepatiques. TIPS *vs* sclerotherapy + propranolol in the prevention of variceal bleeding: preliminary results of a multicenter randomized trial [abstract]. *Hepatology* 1995;22 (Suppl. 297A).
17. Van Buuren HR. *Studies in portal hypertension*. Rotterdam: Erasmus Medical Centre; 2002 (thesis).
18. Papatheodoridis GV, Goulis J, Leandro G, Patch D, Burroughs AK. Transjugular intrahepatic portosystemic shunt compared with endoscopic treatment for prevention of variceal rebleeding: A meta-analysis. *Hepatology* 1999; 30: 612-22.
19. Luca A, D'Amico G, La Galla R, Midiri M, Morabito A, Pagliaro L. TIPS for prevention of recurrent bleeding in patients with cirrhosis: meta-analysis of randomized clinical trials. *Radiology* 1999; 212: 411-21.
20. Burroughs AK, Vangeli M. Transjugular intrahepatic portosystemic shunt *versus* endoscopic therapy: randomized trials for secondary prophylaxis of variceal bleeding: an updated meta-analysis. *Scand J Gastroenterol* 2002; 37: 249-52.
21. Meddi P, Merli M, Lionetti R, De Santis A, Valeriano V, Masini A, et al. Cost analysis for the prevention of variceal rebleeding: a comparison between transjugular intrahepatic portosystemic shunt and endoscopic sclerotherapy in a selected group of Italian cirrhotic patients. *Hepatology* 1999; 29: 1074-7.
22. Barange K, Peron JM, Imani K, Otal P, Payen JL, Rousseau H, et al. Transjugular intrahepatic portosystemic shunt in the treatment of refractory bleeding from ruptured gastric varices. *Hepatology* 1999; 30: 1139-43.
23. Chau TN, Patch D, Chan YW, Nagral A, Dick R, Burroughs AK. "Salvage" transjugular intrahepatic portosystemic shunts: gastric fundal compared with esophageal variceal bleeding. *Gastroenterology* 1998; 114: 981-7.
24. Fantin AC, Zala G, Risti B, Debatin JF, Schopke W, Meyenberger C. Bleeding anorectal varices: successful treatment with transjugular intrahepatic portosystemic shunting (TIPS). *Gut* 1996; 38: 932-5.
25. Haskal ZJ, Scott M, Rubin RA, Cope C. Intestinal varices: treatment with the transjugular intrahepatic portosystemic shunt. *Radiology* 1994; 191: 183-7.
26. Johnson PA, Laurin J. Transjugular portosystemic shunt for treatment of bleeding stomal varices. *Dig Dis Sci* 1997; 42: 440-2.
27. Jonnalagadda SS, Quiason S, Smith OJ. Successful therapy of bleeding duodenal varices by TIPS after failure of sclerotherapy. *Am J Gastroenterol* 1998; 93: 272-4.
28. Fitzgerald JB, Chalmers N, Abbott G, Lee SH, Warnes TW, Youngs GR, et al. The use of TIPS to control bleeding caput medusae. *Br J Radiol* 1998; 71: 558-60.
29. Guth E, Katz MD, Hanks SE, Teitelbaum GP, Ralls P, Korula J. Recurrent bleeding from ileal varices treated by transjugular intrahepatic portosystemic shunt: value of Doppler ultrasonography in diagnosis and follow-up. *J Ultrasound Med* 1996; 15: 67-9.
30. Grubel P, Pratt DS, Elhelw T. Transjugular intrahepatic portosystemic shunt for portal decompression before abdominal and retroperitoneal surgery in patients with severe portal hypertension. *J Clin Gastroenterol* 2002; 34: 489-90.
31. Benador N, Grimm P, Lavine J, Rosenthal P, Reznik V, Lemire J. Transjugular intrahepatic portosystemic shunt prior to renal transplantation in a child with autosomal-recessive polycystic kidney disease and portal hypertension: A case report. *Pediatr Transplant* 2001; 5: 210-4.
32. Guglielmi A, Girlanda R, Lombardo F, de Manzoni G, Frameglia M, Pelosi G, et al. TIPS allowing for an endoscopic mucosal resection of early gastric cancer in a cirrhotic patient with severe hypertensive gastropathy: report of a case. *Surg Today* 1999; 29: 902-5.
33. Angeloni S, Merli M, Salvatori FM, De Santis A, Fanelli F, Pepino D, et al. Polytetrafluoroethylene-covered stent grafts for TIPS procedure: 1-year patency and clinical results. *Am J Gastroenterol* 2004; 99: 280-5.

34. Hausegger KA, Karnel F, Georgieva B, Tauss J, Portugaller H, Deutschmann H, *et al.* Transjugular intrahepatic portosystemic shunt creation with the Viatorr expanded polytetrafluoroethylene-covered stent-graft. *J Vasc Interv Radiol* 2004; 15: 239-48.
35. Angermayr B, Cejna M, Koenig F, Karnel F, Hackl F, Gangl A, *et al.* Survival in patients undergoing transjugular intrahepatic portosystemic shunt: ePTFE-covered stentgrafts *versus* bare stents. *Hepatology* 2003; 38: 1043-50.
36. Bureau C, Garcia-Pagan JC, Otal P, Pomier-Layrargues G, Chabbert V, Cortez C, *et al.* Improved clinical outcome using polytetrafluoroethylene-coated stents for TIPS: results of a randomized study. *Gastroenterology* 2004; 126: 469-75.

II

Bilio-pancreatic disorders

Critical appraisal of laparoscopic bile duct exploration

Bertrand Millat

Department of Visceral Surgery, University Hospital Saint Eloi, 34295 Montpellier, France

Laparoscopic exploration of the common bile duct (CBD) is performed either for the diagnosis or the treatment of CBD stones. CBD stones demonstrated by laparoscopic intraoperative cholangiography (IOC), or ultrasonography (LUS), are extracted either through the cystic duct or through choledochotomy. An alternative for the treatment of CBD stones is to perform an endoscopic sphincterotomy (CES) either before, during or after laparoscopic cholecystectomy. The aim of this review is to analyze and to comment the prospective and comparative studies, randomized or not, evaluating these different techniques.

Intraoperative cholangiography

Routine *versus* selective IOC

Two prospective randomized studies [1, 2] have assessed the value of routine intraoperative cholangiography during laparoscopic cholecystectomy. In both trials, pregnancy or allergy to iodinated contrast material were contraindications for IOC. Pre- or intraoperative variables considered as compelling reasons for IOC are reported in *table I*.

• **In the first prospective trial** [1], of 164 consecutive patients undergoing attempted laparoscopic cholecystectomy during ter months, 56 and 59 patients were randomized to the IOC and non-IOC groups, respectively. IOC was unsuccessful in three patients (5.4%) because of avulsion (two patients) or failed intubation (one patient) of the cystic duct. Cholangiograms were obtained using static radiographic techniques. IOC was associated with a mean 16-minute increase in duration (94 ± 3 min *versus* 78 ± 3 min; p < 0.01) and a mean 690-US $ increase in cost of operation. Relevant information was obtained from IOC in eight patients and changed the intraoperative management in four. In one patient, a filling defect was interpreted retrospectively as a 3 mm ductal stone. At one month postoperatively, patients in both groups had normal liver tests and no instances of symptoms related to retained CBD stones were recorded during the two to 12 months follow-up.

Table I. Criteria for routine intraoperative cholangiography

- **Preoperative factors**
  Endoscopic retrograde cholangiography +/- sphincterotomy
  Ultrasonographic findings
    Common bile duct size over 6 mm
    Choledocholithiasis
  History of jaundice or pancreatitis
  Elevated bilirubin, alkaline phosphatase, transaminases

- **Intraoperative factors**
  Unclear anatomy
  Conversion to open cholecystectomy
  Dilated cystic duct over 4 mm

- **In the second trial** [2], 138 and 137 patients from two surgical centers were randomized to the IOC and non-IOC groups, respectively, during 21 months. Two hundred and sixty-two (95.3%) operations were performed laparoscopically. IOC was unsuccessful in 27 (19.6%) patients, most often because of failure to intubate the cystic duct. Contrast material was injected under fluoroscopic control and cholangiograms were obtained using two static images. IOC was associated with a mean 15-minute increase in duration of operation (92 ± 31 min *versus* 77 ± 28 min; $p < 0.01$). Additional financial and logistic expenditures associated with IOC were not reported. Unsuspected cystic or CBD stones were diagnosed by IOC in three patients. A CBD stone was diagnosed by IOC in a fourth patient but nothing was found on postoperative endoscopic retrograde cholangiopancreatography (ERC). None of the patients in the IOC group had any evidence of symptomatic retained stones within the 12-month follow-up period. Five patients had symptomatic retained CBD stones in the non-IOC group and four additional patients had postoperative abnormalities in liver enzymes tests during follow-up. Overall eight ERC were performed postoperatively in the non-IOC group. One biliary injury (clipping of the main hepatic duct) was reported in a patient without IOC, leading to reoperation for bilio-digestive reconstruction.

Techniques of cholangiography

Cholangiograms obtained during laparoscopy are usually performed after catheterization of the cystic duct through a cholangioclamp (Storz Endoscopy-America, Culver-city, California, USA), or inserting a catheter through a hollow gasketed needle pinned through the abdominal wall along the right subcostal margin. Difficulties in catheterization of the small cystic duct have led to consider cholecystocholangiography by direct puncture of the gallbladder as an alternative to cystic duct cholangiography. In a prospective controlled trial of 69 patients [3], cystic duct cholangiography (38 patients) was compared with cholecystocholangiography (31 patients) in a consecutive non randomized fashion. Optimal visualization of the biliary tree was obtained in 29 cases (76%), and seven cases

(22%), respectively. The failure rates were 8% and 52%, respectively. The anatomy of the cystic duct junction was clearly delineated in 34 cases (89.5%) with cystic duct cholangiography and in eleven cases (35.5%) with cholecystocholangiography, respectively. Cystic duct cholangiography revealed unsuspected CBD stones in three cases; however, choledocholithiasis was missed by cholecystocholangiography in at least two patients.

Fluorocholangiography (FIOC), unlike static IOC, allows real-time assessment of the CBD. Furthermore, FIOC allows rapid discrimination between air bubbles and CBD stones and might decrease the risk of false positive IOC. FIOC was attempted in 336 patients undergoing laparoscopic cholecystectomy [4] and was successfully completed in 328 (95%). Reasons for failed FIOC included a perforated or avulsed cystic duct (three patients) and inability to canulate the cystic duct (five patients). No demonstrable morbidity could be attributed to IOC. There were no false-positive and one false-negative (0.3%) FIOC examinations. Of 14 patients with air bubbles during FIOC, only one actually was a stone. CBD stones were discovered by FIOC in 23 patients and cleared laparoscopically in 16 (70%). Abnormal anatomic findings were seen in 35 (11%) of 328 completed IOC but affected operative management in only 3% of patients. When compared with a retrospective group of 56 patients undergoing static IOC [1], FIOC took significantly less time to perform (14 ± 1 min *versus* 24 ± 1 min; $p < 0.001$).

Comments

Cystic duct cholangiography is clearly better than cholecystocholangiography, and fluoroscopic imaging should be the standard for IOC. Until now, no specific clinically significant complications directly attributable to laparoscopic IOC have been reported. Cystic duct perforation or avulsion during an attempted IOC have an uneventful postoperative course. Expected success rates for laparoscopic IOC are in a 90 to 100% range. Inability to canulate a narrow cystic duct is the main cause of failure. The success rate is higher in a group with selective indications for IOC when compared to a group without these same indications, 98% *versus* 93%, respectively [4]. Willingness to succeed as well as the ability to deal with IOC findings laparoscopically [4] are associated with increased success rates. Gentle compression of the CBD under real time fluoroscopic vision with an atraumatic instrument usually discriminates between air bubbles and stones, and enhances visualization of small calculi, as well as adequate filling of the intra- and extra-hepatic ducts [6], with no need for intraoperative drugs (morphine sulfate, glucagon) [1], thus possibly decreasing the false positive rate to less than 1% [4, 6].

In addition to screening for potential, asymptomatic CBD stones, the second all-important attribute of IOC is that it provides adequate definition of ductal anatomy. No clear-cut relationship has been established between anatomical ductal variations and the risk of CBD injuries. Of concern, however, is the reported delay for the diagnosis of iatrogenic bile duct injuries and its impact on increased morbidity. Fifty-one to 78% of bile duct injuries are not diagnosed at the time of operation [7-10]. When performed after clipping (but not cutting) the anatomical structures identified by careful dissection such as the cystic artery and the cystic duct, a correctly interpreted IOC allows the detection of the most frequently reported cause of CBD injury, *i.e.* mistaken identification of a narrow main bile duct in place of the cystic duct. The only severe bile duct injury reported in these trials was an inadvertent clipping of the common hepatic duct requiring reoperation and biliodigestive anastomosis, which occurred in the group of laparoscopic cholecystectomy without IOC [2]. As previously shown [5, 11], the prospective studies analyzed herein [1-4] demonstrate that several pre- or intraoperative variables allow to discriminate a population in whom the risk of CBD stones is less than 2 or 3%. However, just calculating the cost-effectiveness of routine IOC in terms of postoperative treatment of symptomatic retained stones [11] does not tell the whole story. The potential protective effect of IOC regarding the risk of CBD injury has been underlined [12-16]. The disastrous consequences and enormous costs bile duct injuries incur have to be taken in account for evaluation of cost-efficiency of IOC. The rate of bile duct injuries associated with laparoscopic cholecystectomy is approximately 0.6%. The mean estimated life-long costs of treating just one patient with a CBD injury will pay for more than one thousand routine IOC. In all cases associated with an increased risk of CBD injury, and particularly during the first 20 to 30 cases of laparoscopic cholecystectomy, IOC should be mandatory. Ability to perform an IOC, not just removing the gallbladder, should be one of the requirements for adequate training in laparoscopic biliary surgery.

Laparoscopic ultrasonography (LUS)

Several studies on LUS have been published [17-29]. Overall, conclusions of these studies favor LUS as compared to IOC: LUS is performed with a higher success rate, in less time, with better specificity, but with less precision with regard to the delineation of biliary tree anatomy. LUS is of little, if any, help in the diagnosis or prevention of bile duct injuries. However, some methodological limitations challenge this general, favourable opinion. Many of the papers report on small samples of patients with CBD stones and none of these studies fully correspond to appropriate methodological criteria for evaluation of diagnostic methods: no comparison *vis-à-vis* one undebatable gold standard, discrepancies between the number of retrieved stones by exploration and the number of stones diagnosed by one or the other methods under investigation, interpretation of IOC *versus* LUS not blinded and no mention of the follow-up period to ensure the false negative rate except for one study [22] where it was 5.4 months.

The population studied in series [20, 22, 23, 25-27] in which at least ten patients had stones is one in whom patients with suspected stones had preoperative ERCP [20, 23, 25, 26]. Sensitivity of IOC was equal or better than that of LUS in four out of six studies [22, 25-27]. LUS was used as the "gold standard" in the study reporting the lower sensitivity [23] for IOC. LUS cannot detect the passage into the duodenum of contrast material, as does IOC.

Comments

LUS is operator-dependent, as shown by the wide range of time necessary to accomplish this investigation in one multicenter study [23], and obviously there is a learning curve (20 to 40 examinations), which might be difficult to obtain in small volume centers where the 10% prevalence of CBD stones means that the learning curve may take one to two years to reach.

While detection of smaller stones by LUS should increase its sensitivity, most of these stones are reputed to be flushed out through the sphincter and therefore the question arises if such small stones require any treatment at all. Specificity of LUS is higher (less false positives) than of IOC. When IOC and LUS were combined, there were less than 1% of false-positives [23-27] and surgical exploration was not performed in any of these patients. The question that comes to mind is whether LUS should be a screening test, and IOC performed only in case of doubt or should IOC be the screening test, and LUS used only when IOC is of doubtful value?

IOC performs better than LUS to delineate the entire biliary tree, from the intrahepatic tree to the pancreatic portion of the CBD [22, 23, 26]. Injection of saline into the biliary tree enhanced the images obtained by LUS [22], especially in the distal portion of the bile duct. In the only study in favouring of LUS as regards anatomical delineation [20], LUS was performed by one operator only, raising the question of generalization of the method. LUS is usually performed before any dissection, and therefore before any iatrogenic injury could occur.

Laparoscopic extraction of common bile duct stones

Once detected during laparoscopic IOC, laparoscopic extraction of CBD stones is a logical extension of the procedure. Laparoscopic exploration of the CBD can be performed either through the cystic duct or by laparoscopic choledochotomy. A critical evaluation of the retrospective and prospective series on laparoscopic CBD exploration published since 1989 shows that both procedures are feasible and safe [30]. Any comparisons between the two techniques would be fallacious because of their obviously different indications. Nonetheless, whenever feasible, laparoscopic transcystic CBD exploration best fulfills the expectancies of a mini-invasive approach. Laparoscopic management of CBD stones is considered as technically difficult and demanding, requiring advanced laparoscopic skills as well as expensive endoscopic and radiological equipment. Endoscopic sphincterotomy (ES) is commonly proposed preoperatively as *the* alternative to surgery for CBD stones. ES is indicated in patients with severe cholangitis [31-34] for urgent drainage of infected bile, and in patients with retained stones after cholecystectomy. In open conventional surgery, controlled studies have not shown that ES, performed either prior to surgery [35-38] or in patients with gallbladder *in situ* [39,40], was superior to single-step surgical management. Conclusions reached by these randomized trials have not been extrapolated to laparoscopic biliary surgery.

Two additional randomized trials have been performed, comparing ES either before [41, 42] or after [43] laparoscopic cholecystectomy, *versus* the single-stage laparoscopic management in patients with CBD stones. Although not directly addressing the laparoscopic treatment of CBD stones, a third trial has compared ERC before or after laparoscopic cholecystectomy with IOC in patients with suspected CBD stones [44].

As concerns the EAES (European Association for Endoscopic Surgery) multicenter prospective randomized controlled trial, both preliminary findings [41] and final results [42] comparing endoscopic stone extraction followed by laparoscopic cholecystectomy

(Group A) *versus* laparoscopic cholecystectomy with CBD exploration (Group B) were published. The preliminary analysis was carried out on 207 randomized patients while the final analysis involved 300 patients, including 31 (10%) with protocol violations. Preoperative work-up leading to suspicion of CBD stones was highly accurate with 75.3% and 80% of patients having confirmed CBD stones in groups A and B, respectively. Overall, stones were demonstrated in 110 of 153 (72%) patients selected for ERC. Seven of 153 ERC failed, for a 95.4% success rate. Endoscopic stone extraction was successful in 93 of 109 (85%) attempts. The total number of endoscopic procedures performed to achieve complete CBD clearance in the 93 patients was not reported in the final analysis [42]. In group B, stones were demonstrated in 110 of 139 (79%) diagnostic IOC. One of 171 diagnostic or pre-therapeutic IOC failed, for a success rate of 99.4%. Laparoscopic CBD stone extraction was attempted in 134 patients and was successful in 110 (82%). Nineteen patients were converted to open surgery for ductal stone clearance and five patients underwent successful postoperative ES. Including patients with protocol violations, the conversion rates to open surgery were 6% (9 of 150) and 12% (18 of 150) in groups A and B, respectively (p = 0.08). Five of the 9 and 14 of the 18 conversions were performed for unsuccessful ductal stone clearance. The success rates of transcystic and laparoscopic CBD explorations were 79% and 82%, respectively (p = 0.67). There were no significant differences between the two groups regarding the minor and major postoperative complication rates. Patients with single-stage surgical treatment (Group B) were in hospital for three days less than patients in group A (two-stage management) (median, 6.0 days, 25-75% Inter Quartile Range = 4.25-12 *versus* median, 9.0 days, 25-75% Inter Quartile Range 5.5-14; p < 0.05).

Postoperative ERC-ES is an alternative to laparoscopic exploration of the CBD [43] when ductal stones have been demonstrated by laparoscopic IOC. During a 24-month period, 427 of 471 patients (91%) undergoing laparoscopic cholecystectomy were considered to have a satisfactory IOC, among which 80 (17%) were found to have CBD stones. Among 40 patients randomized to laparoscopic CBD exploration, 30 (75%) had their ducts cleared at the time of surgery, either by the transcystic route (23 patients) or by a laparoscopic choledochotomy (seven patients). Nine patients required postoperative ERC-ES and one was converted to open surgery. Final duct clearance in this group was 100%. Morbidity occurred in six patients. Complete clearance was achieved in 37 of 40 (93%) patients randomized to postoperative ERC-ES. Thirty patients had one, five patients had two and two patients had three endoscopic procedures. Two patients had a biliary stent after a failed second ES and one patient had CBD stones left *in situ*. Three patients experienced bleeding after ES. Including postoperative ERC, conversions to open surgery and reoperations as additional procedures, a total of 52 procedures were performed to achieve a 100% ductal clearance in the first group while 94 procedures were necessary to achieve a 93% ductal clearance in the second group. Hospital stay, including all readmissions, was shorter (p < 0.001) after laparoscopic CBD exploration (median 1 day, range 1-26) than after postoperative ERC-ES (median 3.5 days, range 1-11). In patients for whom the first ERC failed to clear the CBD, ERC was repeated one week later.

A prospective randomized trial [44] has compared pre- *versus* postoperative ERC-ES in 59 patients with suspected or demonstrated CBD stones because of a mild pancreatitis. As acute pancreatitis itself is a poor marker of CBD stones [45], additional variables leading to suspicion of persisting CBD stones were used as inclusion criteria: CBD size greater than 7 mm on admission ultrasound, serum total bilirubin greater than 1.7 mg/dL. Routine laparoscopic IOC for ductal anatomy clarification was a policy of the surgical team regardless of protocol requirements. CBD stones were found in 12 of 30 patients (40%) randomized to routine preoperative ERC. Stone retrieval was successful in 11 of the 12 ES. The last patient sustained post-ERC pancreatitis complicating failed ductal clearance. All 30 patients underwent successful laparoscopic cholecystectomy and no additional CBD stones were found on IOC. Twenty-nine patients were randomized to laparoscopic cholecystectomy without routine preoperative ERC. Eight of 28 patients with successful IOC had CBD stones and seven underwent postoperative therapeutic ERC with ES and stone extraction. One patient with CBD stones on IOC had a choledochoduodenal fistula prompting conversion to open surgery. Overall, nine diagnostic ERC and seven ES were performed in this group. Mean hospital stay was significantly longer and mean total cost was significantly higher in the preoperative as compared with the postoperative ERC group, 11.7 *versus* 9 days and 9,426 *versus* 7,798 US $, respectively.

Comments

Diagnostic and therapeutic choices in cholelithiasis must be considered conjointly. Data gathered from randomized trials have demonstrated that ES, as an additional procedure to surgery, does not improve the clinical results in patients fit for primary single-stage surgical treatment, whether performed laparoscopically or not. Discussions regarding the optimal way to treat patients with demonstrated CBD stones could lead to endless debate. Due to marginal differences between the endoscopic and surgical techniques, the number of patients needed to show any significant difference in terms of morbidity, mortality or clearance rates would be enormous and therefore unrealistic. Cholangitis, jaundice, and CBD stones, as demonstrated on percutaneous ultrasonography, are the only reliable preoperative indicators available with predictive value of CBD stones better than 50% [45]. Severe cholangitis is an unquestionable indication for urgent endoscopic drainage, regardless of whether the CBD can be cleared of associated stones or not [31].

The notorious insufficiencies of all other preoperative indicators for CBD stones should lead to a requiem for preoperative invasive diagnostic procedures, both in terms of risk-benefits and costs.

All surgeons undertaking laparoscopic cholecystectomy must be able to perform an IOC. When IOC demonstrates CBD stones, appropriate treatment is decided according to available equipment and skills. Transcystic clearance of CBD stones is successful in at least two of three patients [30]. In case of large (more than 20 mm) stones or other potential difficulties as regards postoperative ES such as a periampullary diverticulum [43], conversion to open surgery is indicated in case of failed laparoscopic CBD exploration. In the other cases, the available data [43, 44] do not allow any formal conclusions regarding the alternative between advanced laparoscopic biliary explorations and postoperative ES. The potential risk of reoperation in case of failed postoperative ES might be more theoretical than practical [44]. In one decision analysis [46], assessing different approaches to using ERC in patients undergoing laparoscopic cholecystectomy, postoperative ERC was associated with less costs and morbidity, but laparoscopic CBD exploration was not considered in the study design. Last, before embarking on a more invasive laparoscopic CBD exploration policy for small stones, irretrievable by the transcystic approach, surgeons must remember that asymptomatic migration does exist, even if the definitive fate of small CBD stones remains unknown at the present time. The potential security afforded by temporary biliary drainage still has to be balanced with its unavoidable morbidity [47-49].

References

1. Soper NJ, Dunnegan DL. Routine *versus* selective intra-operative cholangiography during laparoscopic cholecystectomy. *World J Surg* 1992; 16: 1133-40.
2. Nies C, Bauknecht F, Groth C, Clerici T, Bartsch D, Lange J, Rothmund M. Intraoperative cholangiographie als routinemethod? Eine prospektive, kontrollierte, randomisierte studie. *Chirurg* 1997; 68: 892-7.
3. Glättli A, Mtezger A, Klaiber C, Maddern GJ, Baer HU. Cholecystocholangiography *vs* cystic duct cholangiography during laparoscopic cholecystectomy. *Surg Endosc* 1994; 8: 299-301.
4. Jones DB, Dunnegan DL, Soper NJ. Results of a change to routine fluorocholangiography during laparoscopic cholecystectomy. *Surgery* 1995; 118: 693-702.
5. Hauer-Jensen M, Karesen R, Nygaard K, Solheim K, Amlie EJB, Havig O, Rosseland AR. Prospective randomized study of routine intraoperative cholangiography during open cholecystectomy: long-term follow-up and multivariate analysis of predictors of choledocholithiasis. *Surgery* 1993; 113: 318-23.
6. Millat B, Deleuze A, de Saxce B, de Seguin C, Fingerhut A. Routine intraoperative cholangiography is feasible and efficient during laparoscopic cholecystectomy. *Hepato-Gastroenterology* 1997; 44: 22-7.
7. Richardson MC, Bell G, Fullarton GM. Incidence and nature of bile duct injuries following laparoscopic cholecystectomy: an audit of 5,913 cases. West of Scotland Laparoscopic Cholecystectomy Audit Group. *Br J Surg* 1996; 83: 1356-60.
8. Gigot JF, Navez B, Etienne J, Cambier E, Jadoul P, Guiot P, Kestens PJ. A stratified intraoperative surgical strategy is mandatory during laproscopic common bile duct exploration for common bile duct stones. Lessons and limits from an initial experience of 92 patients. *Surg Endosc* 1997; 11: 722-8.
9. Bingham J, McKie LD, McLoughlin J, Diamond T. Biliary complications associated with laparoscopic cholecystectomy: analysis of common misconceptions. *Br J Surg* 2000; 87: 362-73.
10. Mirza DF, Narsimhan KL, FerrazNeto BH, Mayer AD, McMaster P, Buckels JA. Bile duct injury following laparoscopic cholecystectomy: referal pattern and management. *Br J Surg* 1997; 84: 786-90.
11. Sahai AV, Mauldin PD, Marsi V, Hawes RH, Hoffman BJ. Bile duct stones and laparoscopic cholecystectomy: a decision analysis to assess the roles of intraoperative cholangiography, EUS, and ERCP. *Gastrointest Endosc* 1999; 49: 334-43.
12. Woods MS, Traverso LW, Kozarek RA, Tsao J, Rossi RL, Gough D, Donohue JH. Biliary tract complications of laparoscopic cholecystectomy are detected more frequently with routine intraoperative cholangiography. *Surg Endosc* 1995; 9: 1076-80.
13. Kullman E, Borch K, Lindström E, Svanvik J, Anderberg B. Value of routine intraoperative cholangiography in detecting aberrant bile ducts and bile duct injuries during laparoscopic cholecystectomy. *Br J Surg* 1996; 83: 171-5.
14. Stuart SA, Simpson TIG, Alvord LA, Williams MD. Routine intraoperative laparoscopic cholangiography. *Am J Surg* 1998; 176: 632-7.
15. Fletcher DR, Hobbs MST, Tan P, Valinsky LJ, Hockey RL, Pikora TJ, Knuiman MW, Sheiner HJ, Edis A. Complications of cholecystectomy: risks of the laparoscopic approach and protective effects of operative cholangiography. A population based study. *Ann Surg* 1999; 229: 449-57.

16. Huguier M, Bornet P, Charpak Y, Houry S, Chastang C. Selective contraindications based on multivariate analysis for operative cholangiography in biliary lithiasis. *Surg Gynecol Obstet* 1991; 172: 470-4.
17. Greig TD, John TG, Mahadaven M, Garden OJ. Laparoscopic ultrasonography in the evaluation of biliary tree during laparoscopic cholecystectomy. *Br J Surg* 1994; 81: 1202-6.
18. Orda R, Sayfan J, Levy Y. Routine laparoscopic ultrasonography in biliary surgery. *Surg Endosc* 1994; 8: 1239-42.
19. Röthlin MA, Schlumpf R, Largiader F. Laparoscopic sonography. An alternative to routine intraoperative cholangiography? *Arch Surg* 1994; 129: 694-700.
20. Röthlin MA, Schöb O, Schlumpf R, Largiader F. Laparoscopic ultrasonography during cholecystectomy. *Br J Surg* 1996; 83: 1512-6.
21. Pietrabissa A, Di Candio G, Giulanotti PC, Shimi SM, Cuschieri A. Comparative evaluation of contact ultrasonography and transcystic cholangiography during laparoscopic cholecystectomy: a prospective study. *Arch Surg* 1995; 130: 110-4.
22. Barteau JA, Castro D, Arregui ME, Tetik C. A comparison of intraoperative ultrasound *versus* cholangiography in the evaluation of the common bile duct during laparoscopic cholecystectomy. *Surg Endosc* 1995; 9: 490-6.
23. Stiegman GV, Soper NJ, Filipi CJ, McIntyre RC, Callery MP, Cordova JF. Laparoscopic ultrasonography as compared with static or dynamic cholangiography at laparoscopic cholecystectomy. *Surg Endosc* 1995; 9: 1269-73.
24. Thompson DM, Arregui ME, Tetik C, Madden MT, Wegener M. A comparison of laparoscopic ultrasound with digital fluorocholangiography for detecting choledocholithiasis during laparoscopic cholecystectomy. *Surg Endosc* 1998; 12: 929-32.
25. Birth M, Ehlers KU, Delinikolas K, Weiser HF. Prospective randomized comparison of laparoscopic ultrasonography using a flexible-tip ultrasound probe and intraoperative dynamic cholangiography during laparoscopic cholecystectomy. *Surg Endosc* 1998; 12: 30-6.
26. Catheline JM, Turner R, Rizk N, Barrat C, Buenos P, Champault G. Evaluation of the biliary tree during laparoscopic cholecystectomy: laparoscopic ultrasound *versus* intraoperative cholangiography: a prospective study of 150 cases. *Surg Laparosc Endosc* 1998; 8: 85-91.
27. Siperstein A, Pearl J, Macho J, Hansen P, Gitomrsky A, Rogers S. Comparison of laparoscopic ultrasonography and fluorocholangiography in 300 patients undergoing laparoscopic cholecystectomy. *Surg Endosc* 1999; 13: 113-7.
28. Falcone RA, Fegelman EJ, Nussbaum MS, Brown DL, Bebbe TM, Merhar GL, Johannigman JA, Luchette FA, Davis, Jr. K, Hurst JM. A prospective comparison of laparoscopic ultrasound *vs* intraoperative cholangiogram during laparoscopic cholecystectomy. *Surg Endosc* 1999; 13: 784-8.
29. Machi J, Tateishi T, Oishi AJ, Furumoto NL, Oishi RH, Uchida S, Sigel B. Laparoscopic ultrasonography *versus* operative cholangiography during laparoscopic cholecystectomy: review of the literature and a comparison with open intraperative ultrasonography. *J Am Coll Surg* 1999; 188: 360-7.
30. Memon MA, Hassaballa H, Memon MI. Laparoscopic common bile duct exploration: the past, the present, and the future. *Am J Surg* 2000; 179: 309-15.
31. Lai ECS, Mok FPT, Tan ESY, Lo CM, Fan ST, You KT. Endoscopic biliary drainage for severe acute cholangitis. *N Engl J Med* 1992; 326: 1582-6.
32. Neoptolemos JP, Carr-Locke DL, London NJ, Bailey IA, James D, Fossard DP. Controlled trial of urgent endoscopic retrograde cholangiopancreatography and endoscopic sphincterotomy *versus* conservative treatment for acute pancreatitis due to gallstones. *Lancet* 1988; 2: 979-83.
33. Fan ST, Lai ECS, Mok FPT, Lo CML, Zheng SS, Wong J. Early treatment of acute biliary pancreatitis by endoscopic papillotomy. *N Engl J Med* 1993; 328: 228-32.
34. Fölsch UR, Nitsche R, Lüdtke R, Hilgers RA, Creutzfeld W, and the German Study Group on Acute Biliary Pancreatitis. Early ERCP and papillotomy compared with conservative treatment for acute biliary pancreatitis. *N Engl J Med* 1997; 336: 237-42.

35. Neoptolemos JP, Carr-Locke DL, Fossard DP. Prospective randomised study of preoperative endoscopic sphincterotomy *versus* surgery alone for common bile duct stones. *Br Med J* 1987; 294: 470-4.
36. Stain SC, Chohen H, Tsuishoyasha M, Donovan AJ. Choledocolithiasis endoscopic sphincterotomy or common bile duct exploration. *Ann Surg* 1991; 213: 627-34.
37. Stiegman GV, Goff JS, Mansour A, Pearlman N, Reveille RM, Norton L. Precholecystectomy endoscopic cholangiography and stone removal is not superior to cholecystectomy, cholangiography and common duct exploration. *Am J Surg* 1992; 163: 227-30.
38. Suc B, Escat J, Cherqui D, Fourtanier G, Hay JM, Fingerhut A, Millat B. Surgery *vs* endoscopy as primary treatment in symptomatic patients with suspected common bile duct stones. A multicenter prospective randomised trial. *Arch Surg* 1998; 133: 702-8.
39. Hammarström LE, Holmin T, Stridbeck H, Ihse I. Long-term follow-up of a prospective randomized study of endoscopic *versus* surgical treatment of bile duct calculi in patients with gallbladder *in situ*. *Br J Surg* 1995; 82: 1516-21.
40. Targarona EM, Ayuso RMP, Bordas JM, Ros E, Pros I, Martinez J, Teres J, Trias M. Randomised trial of endoscopic sphincterotomy with gallbladder left *in situ versus* open surgery for common bileduct calculi in high-risk patients. *Lancet* 1996; 347: 926-9.
41. European Association of Endoscopic Surgeons (EAES) Ductal Stone Cooperative Group: Cuschieri A, Croce E, Faggioni A, Jakimowicz JJ, Lacy A, Lezoche E, Morino M, Ribeiro VM, Toouli J, Visa J, Wayand W. EAES ductal stone study. Preliminary findings of multi-center prospective randomized trial comparing two-stage *vs* single-stage management. *Surg Endosc* 1996; 10: 1130-5.
42. Cuschieri A, Lezoche E, Morino M, Croce E, Lacy A, Toouli J, Faggioni A, Ribeiro VM, Jakimowicz JJ, Visa J, Hanna GB. EAES multicenter prospective randomized trial comparing two-stage *vs* single-stage management of patients with gallstone disease and ductal calculi. *Surg Endosc* 1999; 13: 952-7.
43. Rhodes M, Sussman L, Cohen L, Lewis MP. Randomized trial of laparoscopic extraction of common bile duct *versus* postoperative endoscopic retrograde cholangiography for common bile duct stones. *Lancet* 1998; 351: 159-61.
44. Chang L, Lo S, Stabile BE, Lewis RJ, Toosie K, de Virgilio C. Preoperative *versus* postoperative endoscopic retrograde cholangiopancreatography in mild to moderate gallstone pancreatitis. A prospective randomized trial. *Ann Surg* 2000; 231: 82-7.
45. Abboud PAC, Malet PF, Berlin JA, Staroscik R, Cabana MD, Clarke JR, Shea JA, Schwartz JS, Williams SV. Predictors of common bile duct stones prior to cholecystectomy: a meta-analysis. *Gastrointest Endosc* 1996; 44: 450-9.
46. Erickson RA, Carlson B. The role of endoscopic retrograde cholangiopancreatography in patients with laparoscopic cholecystectomies. *Gastroenterology* 1995; 109: 252-63.
47. Gharaibeh KI, Heiss HA. Biliary leakage following T-tube removal. *Int Surg* 2000 ; 85: 57-63.
48. Millat B, Atger J, Deleuze A, Briandet H, Fingerhut A, Guillon F, Marrel E, De Seguin C, Soulier P. Laparoscopic treatment for choledocholithiasis: a prospective evaluation in 247 consecutive unselected patients. *Hepatogastroenterology* 1997; 44: 28-34.
49. Moreaux J. Traditional surgical management of common bile duct stones: a prospectivestudy during a 20-year experience. *Am J Surg* 1995; 169: 220-6.

Management of bleeding from the papilla of Vater

D.J. Gouma

Academic Medical Center, Department of Surgery, Amsterdam, The Netherlands

Bleeding from the Papilla of Vater is a relative rare condition which may be difficult to recognize but should be considered in all patients with (upper) gastro-intestinal bleeding of unknown origin.

It includes bleeding originating from the biliary tract, so called haemobilia, as well as bleeding from the pancreatic duct, hemosuccus pancreaticus. A third group consists of patients with a bleeding from the papilla shortly after previous intervention, in particular after endoscopic sphincterotomy and/or biopsy. The clinical symptoms, aetiology, diagnostic procedures and therapeutic options will be discussed.

Clinical presentation

The clinical presentation generally depends on the source of origin and the severity of the bleeding ranging from a pulsative bleed from the papilla leading to melaena, haematemesis and shock to continuous minimal bloodloss leading to anaemia. A recurrent limited bleeding, the so-called "sentinel bleed", is frequently found in both conditions, haemobilia and hemosuccus pancreaticus.

In patients who underwent previous liver or pancreatic surgery combined GI bleeding and bleeding from intra-abdominal drains may occur.

Patients with haemobilia frequently present with a trial of symptoms including abdominal pain, upper GI bleeding and jaundice. In some patients, this is associated with fever and chills due to the cholangitis.

Patients with hemosuccus pancreaticus generally have a more severe bleeding and most patients suffer from acute and chronic pancreatitis with abdominal and radiated back pain. Although biliary obstruction is uncommon, it might also occur in patients with a bleeding from a pseudo-aneurysm in the pancreatic head area or a bleeding located in a pre-existent pancreatic pseudocyst.

Bleeding after endoscopic intervention, most frequently observed after sphincterotomy, generally will occur within 24-48 hours after the procedure and is excluded from further discussion. An urgent re-endoscopy (with local injection therapy) or with subsequent radiological embolisation and in case of failure surgical treatment is indicated.

Aetiology

The most common cause of haemobilia is iatrogenic nowadays, mainly after a percutaneous transhepatic biliary drainage procedure or after liver biopsy. In a recent review, Green et al., reported iatrogenic origin in 70% of the cases in stead of 20% reported from earlier studies [1, 2]. In the same time period the percentage of haemobilia due to trauma decreased from 50% towards 5% [1-3]. The other less frequent causes of haemobilia including an inflammatory origin such as acute cholecystitis and stone erosion in the cystic or hepatic artery as well as a malignant origin, frequently associated with obstructive jaundice, are summarized in table I.

Table I. The aetiology of patients presenting with haemobilia

• **Iatrogenic:**
  – percutaneous transhepatic biliary drainage
  – percutaneous liver biopsy
  – cholecystectomy (with a bile duct injury)
  – liver resection (including Klatskin tumors)
• **Trauma**
• **Inflammation:**
  – acute cholecystitis
  – cholangitis
  – stone erosion in cystic or hepatic artery
	• **Malignancy/tumors:**
	  – cholangiocarcinoma
	  – papillomatosis, cystadenoma, adenoma
	  – HCC
	  – metastasis
	• **Vascular:**
	  – aneurysm (hepatic artery)
	  – pseudoaneurysm

Recently case histories of haemobilia have been published from patients after a bile duct injury presenting initially with sepsis due to bile leakage and subsequent bleeding from the (right) hepatic artery [4]. These patients frequently also will present with an intraabdominal bleeding or a bleeding from the percutaneous transhepatic drainage catheter.

Hemosuccus pancreatitis generally occurs in patients with pancreatitis with inflammation and erosion of one of the pancreatic arteries, most frequently a branch of the splenic artery. However, bleeding from the gastroduodenal artery as well as bleeding from the superior mesenteric artery have also been described. Digestion of the wall of the artery, induced by activation of pancreatic enzymes due to inflammation probably plays a role in this process [5]. Another cause of bleeding from the papilla is described in patients with previous duodenum preserving pancreatic surgery for chronic pancreatitis but the bleeding in these patients will generally also occur from the pancreaticojejunostomy into the lumen as more frequently described in patients after pancreatoduodenectomy [6].

Diagnostic strategy

Many patients will present with the so-called "sentinel bleed" a few days before a second more severe bleeding and frequently no diagnostic procedures are performed at that stage and the importance of this clinical phenomenon is not recognized. In other patients multiple endoscopic diagnostic procedures have been performed previously for unrecognized gastrointestinal bleeding.

Upper GI endoscopy should be the first procedure to exclude the more common other causes of bleeding. Erythrocyte scans have been used in the past but have limited value to identify the exact location of the bleeding and are frequently false negative. If blood is seen at the origin of the papilla urgent further investigation is warranted.

For hemodynamically stable patients without severe active bleeding a contrast enhanced CT scan should be performed to identify a (pseudo) aneurysm. It also may show abnormalities within the liver, haemobilia (blood clot) in the ducts as well as pseudocysts or other abnormalities in the pancreas, or liver, and pancreatitis.

In most patients, angiography may be the next step not only to identify the exact location but also to provide information of the possibility for treatment by arterial embolization and/or stenting of the bleeding site. Most bleedings will be located at the splenic artery and hepatic (gastroduodenal) artery. However, if findings at these locations are negative, the mesenteric artery should also be visualized.

Treatment

The management has been changed radically during the past decade.

Previously surgery was the treatment of choice with ligation of the artery, including the hepatic artery or splenic artery [1, 2]. If not successful and depending on the cause of origin, an urgent cholecystectomy, (hemi) hepatectomy or pancreatic resection may be performed.

More recently, arterial embolization and/or stenting of the affected artery has been introduced, a relative minimal invasive procedure to obtain hemostasis in particular in patients with pseudo-aneurysm. A success rate between 3% and 79% has been reported [6].

Embolisation is generally performed for a bleeding from the gastro-duodenal artery or hepatic artery side branches from the mesenteric. Stenting by a covered stent is performed for a bleeding from the mesenteric artery or hepatic artery.

In patients who underwent previous surgery and suffering from sepsis due to leakage of an anastomosis and severe bleeding, surgery might be indicated for management of the intra-abdominal infections ; however, even in these cases embolization could be helpful as a temporary measurement stabilizing the patients for surgery [7, 8]. Embolization and stenting in patients with acute pancreatitis or infection/abscess does have a higher risk for rebleeding.

Arterial embolization stenting is associated with lower morbidity and mortality than surgery and should therefore be considered in all patients as first choice treatment.

The management of these patients, frequently requiring urgent intervention, is mainly dependant on local expertise and a multi-disciplinary approach is warranted

References

1. Sandblom Ph. *Haemobilia*. C.C. Thomas, Springfield: 1972.
2. Green MH, Duell RM, Johnson CD, Jamieson NV. Haemobilia. *Br J Surg* 2001; 88: 773-86.
3. Rousseau A, Regimbeau JM, Vibert E, Vullierme MP, Sauvanet A, Belghiti J. Haemobilia after blunt hepatic trauma: a sometimes delayed complication. *Ann Chir* 2004; 129: 41-5.
4. Journe S, De Simone P, Laureys M, Le Moine O, Gelin M, Closset J. Right hepatic artery pseudoaneurysm and cystic duct leak after laparoscopic cholecystectomy. *Surg Endosc* 2004; 18: 554-6.
5. Sakorafas GH, Sarr MG, Farley DR, Que FG, Andrews JC, Farnell MB. Hemosuccus pancreaticus complicating chronic pancreatitis: an obscure upper gastrointestinal bleeding. *Langenbecks Arch Surg* 2000; 385: 124-8.
6. Otah E, Cushin BJ, Rozenblit GN, Neff R, Otah KE, Cooperman AM. Visceral artery pseudoaneurysms following pancreatoduodenectomy. *Arch Surg* 2002; 137: 55-9.
7. Berge Henegouwen MI van, Allema JH, Gulik TM van, Verbeek PC, Obertop H, Gouma DJ. Delayed massive haemorrhage after pancreatic and biliary surgery. *Br J Surg* 1995; 82: 1527-31.
8. Castro SMM de, Kuhlmann KFD, Busch ORC, Delden OM van, Lameris JS, Gulik TM van, Obertop H, Gouma DJ. Delayed massive hemorrhage after pancreatic and biliary surgery: embolization or surgery? *Ann Surg* 2004, in press.

III

Benign GI disorders: basic concepts

New Developments in the Management of Benign GI Disorders.
D.J. Gouma, G.J. Krejs, G.N. Tytgat, Y. Finkel, eds. John Libbey Eurotext, Paris © 2004, pp. 59-68.

Molecular biology for the gastroenterologist

Peter Ferenci

Department of Internal Medicine IV, Gastroenterology and Hepatology, Medical University of Vienna, Austria

The era of genetics began with the observations of Gregor Mendel that changes in the color of flowers and shape of the seeds followed a clear pattern over the years. His fundamental rules of inheritance thus were based on easily recognizable signs. His work preceded the discovery of DNA as carrier of the genetic information. An observed trait is referred to as a **phenotype**; the genetic information defining the phenotype is called the **genotype**. With more advanced understanding of the function of DNA phenotypic genetics were replaced by molecular genetics. In contrast to phenotypic genetics which assumes that gene products are either fully functional or devoid of function as consequence of a mutation molecular genetics describe variations in the base sequence of gene. Such changes are not always associated with impaired functions of the gene product. Even gene products of mutated genes may still have some residual function. Thus, the presence of a change in the base sequence does not necessarily imply the presence of phenotypic disease. These fundamental differences to phenotype based genetics limit the role of molecular genetics in clinical medicine. This review discusses the application of molecular genetics in general with a specific focus on hereditary diseases of the digestive organs *(table I)*.

Definitions

To understand the implications of molecular genetics, several basic definitions are needed.

What constitutes a normal gene?

A normal gene is defined by the base sequence which is observed in the majority of healthy subjects in a given population and is called the **"wild type"**. Definition of "healthy" requires the presence of a functionally normal gene product and the absence of phenotypic

Table I. Selected genetic diseases in gastroenterology and hepatology

Diseases	Gene	References
• **Cholestatic liver diseases**		[29]
– Byler's disease, Summerskill syndrome	FIC1	
– Progressive familial intrahepatic cholestasis-2	ABCB11	
– Progressive familial intrahepatic cholestasis-3	ABCB4	
– Dubin-Johnson syndrome	ABCB2	
• **Hepatic storage diseases**		
– Wilson disease	ATP7B	[30]
– Hemochromatosis	HFE	[31]
• **Colon cancer**		[32]
– Familial polyposis coli	APC	[33]
– Hereditary nonpolyposis colon cancer	MSH2, MLH1	[34, 35]
– Peutz-Jeghers syndrome	STK11	[36]
• **Idiopathic pancreatitis**		
– Cystic fibrosis	CFTR	[2]
– Hereditary pancreatitis	Trypsinogen, SPINK	[37, 38]
• **Crohn's disease**	NOD2	[39, 40]

disease. Base variations of the "wild type" gene in healthy subjects are named "**DNA-polymorphisms**". These alternative forms of a gene or a genetic marker are referred to as **alleles**. Alleles have no apparent effect on gene expression or function. In other instances, these variants may have subtle effects on gene expression, thereby conferring the adaptive advantages associated with genetic diversity. On the other hand, allelic variants may reflect mutations in a gene that clearly alter its function.

What is a mutation?

A mutation is a base sequence which differs from the "wild type" in a patient presenting with a phenotypic disorder but is never observed in healthy subjects. Thus the definition whether this variation in the base sequence is a disease causing mutation requires testing of healthy subjects. Several disease causing mutations may be present within the same gene. The functional consequences of a mutation are manifold. Mutations may result in the complete absence of gene products ("null" mutations) or in proteins devoid of any function. Such mutations are associated with severe diseases occurring at birth or early childhood. They are mostly due to large deletions or insertion in the DNA or to mutations which result in the occurrence of stop codons ("nonsense" mutations) or of frame shifts due to deletion or insertion of one or two or a small number of nucleotides. Some mutations affect messenger RNA splicing mechanisms.

Functional consequences of a mutation

Functionally, mutations can be broadly classified as gain-of-function and loss-of-function mutations. Gain-of-function mutations are typically dominant; that is, they result in phenotypic alterations when a single allele is affected. Inactivating mutations are usually recessive, and an affected individual is homozygous or compound heterozygous (*i.e.*

carrying two different mutant alleles) for the disease-causing mutations. Other mutations result in less pronounced functional consequences. A single amino acid change may result in an altered, but still functional protein. The mutation may affect the tertiary structure of the gene product, its assembly, inactivation, secretion, or conformational stability.

Allelic heterogeneity refers to the fact that different mutations in the same genetic locus can cause an identical or similar phenotype. Inactivating mutations in genes usually show a near-random distribution. Exceptions include a "founder effect", in which a particular mutation that does not affect reproductive capacity can be traced to a single individual; "hot spots" for mutations, in which the nature of the DNA sequence predisposes to a recurring mutation; and localization of mutations to certain domains that are particularly critical for protein function. Allelic heterogeneity creates a practical problem for genetic testing because one must often examine the entire genetic locus for mutations, as these can differ in each patient.

The difficulties to understand the role of mutation can be best described in cystic fibrosis (CF) [1]. Today more than 850 mutations of the CFTR gene were reported. Some mutations like the ΔF508 mutation are common and account for more than 70% of cases of clinically overt CF. Other mutations are rare and occur sometimes in single families. By far, the missense mutations are the most informative class of mutation in the CFTR gene and account for 40% of the CF mutations. These mutations result in major alterations in the structure and function of their encoded protein. Certain clinical predictions can be made from the analysis of the mutations in the CFTR gene. This "genotype-phenotype" analysis explores the feasibility to predict the severity of disease in specified organs from a particular CFTR mutation. With respect to the sweat gland, the sweat chloride concentrations can be predicted reasonably well based on the genotype. Homozygous carriers of severe mutations, like ΔF508, will routinely have severe pancreatic insufficiency.

CFTR mutations may be classified in another way and that is by their molecular consequence. Channel function is mutation specific with five basic classes of mutations recognized [2]. Some mutations result in a complete absence of a functionally intact CFTR protein (class I). Class II refers to those mutant proteins that have blocked in the processing steps. ΔF508 is an example of a protein that is made but that cannot mature properly; and at the end, there is no functional molecule on the apical membrane. Class III refers to mutant proteins that are blocked in regulation; the protein can get to the apical membrane but cannot be opened by cAMP. CFTR-class IV gene mutations result in proteins which can get to the apical membrane, but when they open, their conductance has altered and the amount of chloride ion that can get through the apical membrane has changed. Class V is a combination of different types of mutations that mainly reduce the total amount of functional CFTR protein on the apical membrane due to reduced synthesis; either at the messenger RNA level, or at the protein maturation level. Over all, class IV and V have a milder consequence than the class I-III and do not cause pancreatic insufficiency.

Genetic deficiency of alpha$_1$-antitrypsin provides a prototype for the diseases associated with conformational instability [3]. The most common mutation is the S mutation. In homozygotes plasma alpha$_1$-antitrypsin concentrations are decreased by 40%. This by itself poses a negligible threat to health, but the S variant becomes important if it is coinherited with the more severe Z mutation, which is present in 4% of Northern

Europeans. In homozygotes plasma alpha$_1$-antitrypsin concentrations are decreased by 85%. Consequently, the plasma concentrations of alpha$_1$-antitrypsin in both ZZ homozygotes and SZ compound heterozygotes are insufficient to ensure lifetime protection of the lungs from proteolytic damage, especially in smokers [4, 5]. The low plasma alpha$_1$-antitrypsin concentrations result not from a lack of synthesis but from a blockage of its processing and secretion [6]. The retained alpha$_1$-antitrypsin aggregates in the endoplasmic reticulum of hepatocytes as inclusions that are readily recognizable on periodic acid-Schiff staining. Z mutant of alpha$_1$-antitrypsin forms long polymers in the endoplasmic reticulum of hepatozytes [7] which are resistant to the usual degradative processes [8].

Tools of molecular genetic analysis

Molecular genetics require the visualization of sequence differences directly in DNA. DNA-polymorphisms in coding regions (exons) or noncoding regions of genes [9] are inherited according to the Mendelian rules. The value of highly variable DNA sequences as genetic markers rests on straightforward principles. Every person carries two copies of each chromosome except the sex chromosomes. If a DNA polymorphism is to be useful in analyzing the transmission of the two chromosomes in a family, then the DNA copies at the polymorphic site of the person under study must be different in the two chromosomes. The likelihood that a given person will have different DNA sequences at the polymorphic site directly determines the usefulness of that site in genetic studies. Chromosomal sites at which the DNA sequences can have many alternative forms are thus ideal sites for genetic markers. At these sites, a person is most likely to carry two alternative DNA sequences, accurately marking the two alternative chromosomes. In the human genome, the sites that have the properties most favorable to such extensive variation include a repetition of the same short DNA sequence a variable number of times. Such sequences are called tandem-repeat sequences (microsatellites). A DNA sequence with such variation may be as short as two base pairs or as long as several hundred base pairs. Highly variable sequences of this type are well distributed throughout the length of every human chromosome. When tandemly repeated sequences are replicated during cell division, the number of repeats can change.

Methods to detect DNA – polymorphisms

Restriction fragment length polymorphism (RFLP) analysis

DNA-polymorphisms can be detected by variations in the size of DNA fragments obtained after digestion with restriction enzymes [10, 11]. Restriction enzymes cut DNA-strands at highly specific sites (restriction site). A variation in the nucleotide sequence may result in the loss or the creation of a new restriction site or in the length of the DNA-fragment between existing restriction sites. Thus, the length (and eventually also the number) of the restriction fragment(s) will be different by Southern Blot analysis. The RFLP pattern is specific for every individual tested. Other methods to study DNA-polymorphisms include the detection of the altered mobility of the PCR-product of DNA segment (single-strand conformational polymorphism – SSCP or denaturing gradient gel electrophoresis – DGGE) and WAVE-DNA fragment analysis which is based on temperature-modulated liquid chromatography and a high-resolution matrix. If the gene is unknown, polymorphic markers flanking the unknown gene can be used to construct haplotypes for DNA-linkage analysis. A haplotype refers to a group of alleles that are closely linked together at a genomic locus. Haplotypes are useful for tracking the transmission of genomic segments within families and for detecting evidence of genetic recombination. By employing various restriction enzymes and DNA-probes, multiple RFLP's for a given gene can be obtained. By this approach, both the paternal and the maternal gene can be "reconstructed". If both genes have different allele patterns which are also different within members of the family, the pattern of its inheritance can be traced within the family.

By haplotype analysis inheritance of a disease can be studied even if the gene/and or the mutation are unknown [12]. Precondition is the testing of an index patient (in whom the disease was diagnosed by standard phenotypic criteria) and both of his/her parents. Limitations are the lack of informative allelic markers within the family and the presence of cross-overs within the region of interest. Haplotype analysis is time consuming and can only be applied in selected families. Haplotype analysis is useful to investigate the origin and geographic distribution of a particular mutation [13].

Direct mutation analysis

Direct sequencing

New technologies allow automated sequence analysis of large portions of a gene to detect points mutations, deletions, inversions and other changes in the nucleotide sequence. However, direct sequencing of the whole plays yet no role in clinical medicine. A more practical approach is first to screen the gene of interest for possible mutation by haplotype analysis or by single-strand conformation polymorphism analysis. Those samples showing a shift of one or both bands or unusual haplotypes can then be sequenced to identify the exact mutation. This approach is quite useful as research tool, but impractical for clinical diagnosis.

PCR-based detection of known mutations

A variety of approaches are commonly used to detect mutations. The simplest takes advantage of the base-sequence specificity of restriction endonucleases. These enzymes recognize precise sequences of four to eight bases and cut double-stranded DNA only at these sites. A mutation at such a site will prevent the enzyme from cutting there; conversely, a mutation may result in the creation of a new enzyme-recognition site and lead to cutting where it normally should not occur. To detect the mutation, DNA surrounding the site of potential mutation is amplified by the polymerase chain reaction (PCR), the product is incubated with the restriction enzyme, and then the DNA is analyzed by electrophoresis. If the enzyme cuts, two fragments will result; otherwise there will be a single fragment. The presence or absence of the mutation can be inferred, depending on whether the mutation creates or destroys an enzyme-recognition site.

The other scheme for detecting mutations is based on the specificity of the PCR reaction itself. A PCR primer is designed that ends right at the site of a potential mutation. If the primer is homologous to the wild-type sequence, it will amplify only the wild-type sequence in conjunction with another primer some distance away in the gene. The wild-type primer will not amplify mutant DNA, however. Conversely, a primer that is homologous to the mutant sequence will amplify only mutant DNA. If the PCR is carried out with both sets of primers in separate reactions, the presence or absence of mutant and wild-type sequences can easily be determined. Here multiple sequences can be assayed simultaneously in a single sample, as long as the sizes of the PCR products from each segment differ.

The direct determination of mutations is independent of family analysis. There is no need to test an index patient with the disease. PCR-based mutation assays can be automated and thus allow mass screening. Multiplex PCR-strips can detect the most common mutations of a particular disease simultaneously. Several mutation assays are commercially available now (*i.e.* for cystic fibrosis, hemochromatosis, familial adenomatous polyposis).

Interpretation of test results

Molecular genetic analysis can yield three possible findings: the tested subject is either a homozygous or a heterozygous carrier of the mutation, or does not carry the mutation at all.

Homozygous mutation carrier

Genotypic diagnosis in a healthy subject raises the question whether tested subject will ever develop the disease. In most hereditary diseases, there is no complete penetrance of the disease. In genetic hemochromatosis for example, a large proportion of C282Y (the typical mutation) homozygotes have no evidence of iron overload [14, 15].

Heterozygous mutation carrier

The most important question is, whether the tested subject is (and will remain) free of a disease or not. According to Mendelian rules, subjects carrying a "wild type" and a disease causing gene with autosomal recessive inheritance are healthy. This statement is only valid if the other gene not carrying the mutation is also functionally intact.

Compound heterozygotes

The gene not having the mutation may have a different (disease causing) one, which is not detected by the assay. Such compound heterozygotes may suffer from the disease (diagnosed by phenotypic criteria). Unfortunately this is not an exception but a general rule. In most inherited disease multiple different mutations of the affected gene are present (*i.e.* more than 800 in cystic fibrosis). Mutations may reflect a common ancestor and are enriched in certain populations but may be absent in others.

Haploinsufficiency

Mutation in a single allele can result in a situation in which one normal allele is not sufficient for a normal phenotype. This phenomenon applies, for example, to expression of rate-limiting enzymes in heme synthesis that cause porphyrias. Mutation in a single allele can also result in loss of function due to a dominant-negative effect.

Loss of heterozygosity

Subjects with a normal and an abnormal gene without any apparent disease may undergo somatic mutations of the normal gene later in life. Such event may result in overt dysfunction of the gene product in the affected cells. This loss of heterozygosity is assumed to be one important event in cancerogenesis [16].

Subjects not carrying the mutation

A negative finding does not exclude phenotypic disease, since other mutations of the gene may be present. Furthermore, gene defects may be due to mutation of other genes (*i.e.* mutation of promoters of mismatch repair genes results in hypermethylation of their genes products with impaired functional capacity).

Target populations for molecular genetic testing

Patients with symptomatic phenotypic disease

In patients with hereditary diseases (diagnosed by phenotypic criteria; *i.e.* polyposis coli), DNA analysis strengthens the final diagnosis. In diseases with only few mutations (like in HFE1-associated hemochromatosis), mutation analysis can replace invasive diagnostic tests. In patients with a transferrin saturation index > 45% testing for common HFE1 mutations allows a direct diagnosis of hereditary hemochromatosis. A liver biopsy to ascertain diagnosis is not needed in C282Y homozygotes and C282Y/H63D compound heterozygotes. Due to the large number of mutations in most diseases DNA analysis cannot be used as a diagnostic test.

Another important aspect of mutation analysis is the differentiation of various genetic diseases resulting in similar phenotypic symptoms, like in patients with primary iron overload. Today, at least four independent genetic diseases result in iron accumulation in various organs [17] (HFE1 [chromosome 6p], HFE2 [Hepcidine, chromosome 1q], Ferroportin [chromosome 2q], and Transferrin receptor 2 [chromosome 7q]).

Family screening

Mutation analysis is the state of the art approach for screening the family of index patients and can replace other diagnostic tests to identify subjects at risk to develop the disease. A negative test result in a family member of a patient with a disease-related mutation indicates a low risk of the disease. This can decrease anxiety and, for some diseases, reduce the frequency of monitoring for early signs of the disease.

Population screening

Mutation analysis to detect presymptomatic disease in the general population has not been tested so far. Beyond the discussed difficulties of interpretation of test results several factors limit the use of genetic tests for population screening. First, screening is only appropriate if a validated treatment to prevent occurrence of phenotypic disease is available for asymptomatic subjects. Second, other screening strategies may be more cost effective [18] or straightforward than mutation analysis. For colorectal screening, DNA-based mutation analysis [19] cannot replace endoscopy, since a colonoscopy is needed whether a mutation is present or absent. Furthermore, formation of cancer can be prevented by endoscopic polypectomy. Thus, endoscopy in combination with testing for occult blood in stool [20] will remain the standard for the foreseeable future [21].

Disease association studies

The rapid growth of human genetics creates countless opportunities for studies of disease association. Given the number of potentially identifiable genetic markers and the multitude of clinical outcomes to which these may be linked, the testing and validation of statistical hypotheses in genetic epidemiology is a task of unprecedented scale [22, 23]. The limitations and problems associated with this type of studies was discussed in detail recently [24]. Ideally, selection of candidate genes should be based on biological plausibility [25]. Genes with related pathophysiologic function, those belonging to the same pathway, and those with a biological link between the gene polymorphism studied and the disease should be included. An inaccurate definition of the phenotype can obscure association between a disease subtype and a polymorphism. Moreover, polymorphisms should have a functional significance. Only polymorphisms affecting gene transcription, RNA stability, or splicing or those causing amino acid substitutions are likely to affect protein function. The most common type of genetic variation in humans is the SNP (single nucleotide polymorphism), a stable substitution of a single base, which is found in more than 1% of the population [26]. SNPs are distributed throughout the human genome at an estimated overall frequency of 1 every 1,000 to 2,000 bp.

Association studies are subject to confounding by population stratification if the gene under investigation shows marked variation in allele frequency across subgroups of the population and if these subgroups also differ in their baseline risk of disease [27]. Indeed, population substructure (or admixture) errors can clearly confound case-control study results. For example, factors to be considered in hepatic fibrosis include ethnicity, existence of alcohol abuse, age, menopausal status, use of medication, etc. Meta-analysis of 370 studies addressing 36 genetic associations for various outcomes of disease show that significant between-study heterogeneity (diversity) is frequent, and that the results of the first study correlate only modestly with subsequent research on the same association [28]. The first study often suggests a stronger genetic effect than is found by subsequent studies. Both bias and genuine population diversity might explain why early association studies tend to overestimate the disease protection or predisposition conferred by a genetic polymorphism. In view of countless recent studies investigation genetic associations in disease with multifactorial background and in genetic diseases with low phenotypic penetrance, journals including *Nature Genetics*, *Lancet*, and *Gastroenterology* have set out guidelines for association studies that they wish to publish.

References

1. Noone PG, Knowles MR. "CFTR-opathies": disease phenotypes associated with cystic fibrosis transmembrane regulator gene mutations. *Respir Res* 2001; 2: 328-32.
2. Wilschanski M, Zielinski J, Markiewicz D, *et al.* Correlation of sweat chloride concentration with classes of the cystic fibrosis transmembrane regulator gene mutations. *J Pediatr* 1995; 127: 705-10.
3. Carrell, RW, Lomas DA. Alpha1-antitrypsin deficiency – A model for conformational diseases. *N Engl J Med* 2002; 346: 45-53.
4. Brantly M, Nukiwa T, Crystal RG. Molecular basis of alpha-1-antitrypsin deficiency. *Am J Med* 1988; 84 (Suppl. 6A): 13-31.
5. Turino GM, Barker AF, Brantley ML, *et al.* Clinical features of individuals with PI*SZ phenotype of a_1-antitrypsin deficiency. *Am J Respir Crit Care Med* 1996; 154: 1718-25.
6. Foreman RC, Judah JD, Colman A. Xenopus oocytes can synthesise but do not secrete the Z variant of human a_1-antitrypsin. *FEBS Lett* 1984; 168: 84-8.
7. Elliott PR, Lomas DA, Carrell RW, Abrahams JP. Inhibitory conformation of the reactive loop of a_1-antitrypsin. *Nat Struct Biol* 1996; 3: 676-81.
8. Cabral CM, Choudhury P, Liu Y, Sifers RN. Processing by endoplasmic reticulum mannosidases partitions a secretion-impaired glycoprotein into distinct disposal pathways. *J Biol Chem* 2000; 275: 25015-22.
9. Housman D. Human DNA-polymorphism. *N Engl J Med* 1995; 332: 318-9.
10. Korf B. Molecular Diagnosis (First of 2 parts). *N Engl J Med* 1995; 332: 1218-21.
11. Korf B. Molecular Diagnosis (Second of 2 parts). *N Engl J Med* 1995; 332: 1499-502.
12. Maier-Dobersberger Th, Rack S, Granditsch G, Korninger L, Steindl P, Mannhalter Ch, Ferenci P. Diagnosis of Wilson's disease in an asymptomatic sibling by DNA linkage analysis. *Gastroenterology* 1995; 109: 2015-8.
13. Firneisz G, Lakatos PL, Szalay F, Polli C, Glant TT, Ferenci P. Common Mutations of ATP7B in Wilson Disease Patients from Hungary. *Am J Human Genetics* 2002; 108: 23-8.
14. Crawford DH, Jazwinska EC, Cullen LM, Powell LW. Expression of HLA-linked hemochromatosis in subjects homozygous or heterozygous for the C282Y mutation. *Gastroenterology* 1998; 114: 1003-8.
15. Olynyk JK, Cullen DJ, Aquilia S, Rossi E, Summerville L, Powell LW. A population-based study of the clinical expression of the hemochromatosis gene. *N Engl J Med* 1999; 341: 718-24.
16. Jen J, Kim H, Piantadosi S, *et al.* Allelic loss of chromosome 18q and prognosis in colorectal cancer. *N Engl J Med* 1994; 331: 213-21.
17. Pietrangelo A. Hereditary hemochromatosis. *N Engl J Med* 2004.
18. Hickman PE, Hourigan LF, Powell LW, Cordingley F, Dimeski G, Ormiston B, Shaw J, Ferguson W, Johnson M, Ascough J, McDonell K, Pink A, Crawford DH. Automated measurement of unsaturated iron binding capacity is an effective screening strategy for C282Y homozygous haemochromatosis. *Gut* 2000; 46: 405-9.

19. Traverso G, Shuber A, Levin B, Johnson C, Olsson L, Schoetz DJ Jr, Hamilton SR, Boynton K, Kinzler KW, Vogelstein B. Detection of APC mutations in fecal DNA from patients with colorectal tumors. *N Engl J Med* 2002; 346: 311-20.
20. Rex DK, Johnson DA, Lieberman DA, Burt RW, Sonnenberg A. Colorectal cancer prevention 2000: screening recommendations of the American College of Gastroenterology. *Am J Gastroenterol* 2000; 95: 868-77.
21. Ransohoff DF, Sandler RS. Screening for Colorectal Cancer. *N Engl J Med* 2002; 346: 40-4.
22. McCarthy JJ, Hilfiker R. The use of single-nucleotide polymorphism maps in pharmacogenomics. *Nature Biotechnol* 2000; 18: 505-8.
23. Khoury MJ, Little J. Human genome epidemiology reviews: the beginning of something HuGE. *Am J Epidemiol* 2000; 151: 2-3.
24. Bataller R, North KE, Brenner DA. Genetic polymorphisms and the progression of liver fibrosis: A critical appraisal. *Hepatology* 2003; 37: 493-503.
25. Hirschhorn JN, Lohmueller K, Byrne E, Hirschhorn K. A comprehensive review of genetic association studies. *Genet Med* 2002; 4: 45-61.
26. Syvanen AC. Accessing genetic variation: genotyping single nucleotide polymorphisms. *Nat Rev Genet* 2001; 2: 930-42.
27. Caporaso N. Chapter 4. Selection of candidate genes for population studies. *IARC Sci Publ* 1999; 148: 23-36.
28. Ioannidis JPA, Ntzani EE, Trikalinos TA, Contopoulos-Ioannidis DG. Replication validity of genetic association studies. *Nat Genet* 2001; 29: 306-9.
29. Ferenci P, Zollner F, Trauner M. Hepatic transport systems. *J Gastroenterol Hepatol* 2002; 17: S106-113.
30. Ferenci P. Wilson's disease. *Ital J Gastroenterol Hepatol* 1999; 31: 416-25.
31. Powell LW, Yapp TR. Hemochromatosis. *Clin Liver Dis* 2000; 4: 211-28.
32. Jass JR. Familial colorectal cancer: pathology and molecular characteristics. *Lancet Oncol* 2000; 1: 220-6.
33. Fearnhead NS, Britton MP, Bodmer WF. The ABC of APC. *Hum Mol Genet* 2001; 10: 721-33.
34. Lynch HT, Smyrk T. Hereditary nonpolyposis colorectal cancer (Lynch syndrome). An updated review. *Cancer* 1996; 78: 1149.
35. Wijnen JT, Vasen HF, Khan PM, Zwinderman AH, van der Klift H, Mulder A, Tops C, Moller P, Fodde R. Clinical findings with implications for genetic testing in families with clustering of colorectal cancer. *N Engl J Med* 1998; 339: 511-8.
36. Jenne DE, Reimann H, Nezu J, Friedel W, Loff S, Jeschke R, Muller O, Back W, Zimmer M. Peutz-Jeghers syndrome is caused by mutations in a novel serine threonine kinase. *Nat Genet* 1998; 18: 38-43.
37. Whitcomb DC. Hereditary pancreatitis: new insights into acute and chronic pancreatitis. *Gut* 1999; 45: 317-22.
38. Etemad B, Whitcomb DC. Chronic pancreatitis: diagnosis, classification, and new genetic developments. *Gastroenterology* 2001; 120: 682-707.
39. Hampe J, Cuthbert A, Croucher PJ, Mirza MM, Mascheretti S, Fisher S, Frenzel H, *et al*. Association between insertion mutation in NOD2 gene and Crohn's disease in German and British populations. *Lancet* 2001; 357: 1925-8.
40. Judge T, Lichtenstein GR. The NOD2 gene and Crohn's disease: another triumph for molecular genetics. *Gastroenterology* 2002; 122: 826-8.

Understanding the enteric nervous system

G.E. Boeckxstaens

Division of Gastroenterology and Hepatology, Academic Medical Centre, Amsterdam, The Netherlands

The enteric nervous system (ENS) or the Little Brain of the gut controls gastrointestinal motility and secretion and is involved in visceral sensation. In the last decade, our understanding of the function of the ENS has greatly improved thanks to several interesting discoveries, of which a few were selected.

One of these involves the discovery that the ENS closely interacts with the interstitial cells of Cajal, or the pacemaker cells of the gut. In addition, the importance of the interaction between the ENS and the immune system is now gaining increasing attention. Especially in functional bowel disorders, persistent low grade inflammation after an episode of bacterial gastroenteritis has been suggested to contribute to the development of post-infectious irritable bowel syndrome. Interestingly, also post-operative ileus, a disorder characterised by general gastrointestinal hypomotility, results from the interaction between the immune system and the enteric nervous system. Intestinal manipulation during surgery leads to local inflammation triggering the activation of inhibitory neural pathways. Blockade of the influx of inflammatory cells prevents prolonged ileus and might thus represent a new therapeutic approach to shorten post-operative ileus.

Recently, evidence is also provided that neurons can change their function and phenotype, a phenomenon called neuronal plasticity. Most likely, this mechanism contributes to the development of visceral hypersensitivity, a finding present in more than half of the patients with a functional bowel disorder.

Finally, new developments in stem cell transplantation are briefly discussed as possible new therapeutic approach for disorders characterized by neural loss, such as achalasia.

All these new insights and developments should lead to a better understanding of the ENS, and hopefully to better controlling of the ENS.

The genetic background of gallstone formation

Hermann E. Wasmuth, Siegfried Matern, Frank Lammert

Department of Medicine III, University Hospital Aachen, Aachen University (RWTH), Aachen, Germany

Cholelithiasis is a common disease associated with a substantial economic burden to our health systems. Gallstones are remarkably common in Europe and America, whereas their prevalence is lowest in Africa [1]. In 1976, Brett and Barker calculated the worldwide prevalence of gallstones to be almost 16% based on data of large autopsy studies [2]. These data are confirmed by a recent meta-analysis [3] of 22 ultrasound studies published in the years 1979-1995, which demonstrated the prevalence rate of cholecystolithiasis to be 10-12% in Europe.

Principally there are two major gallstone types, cholesterol and pigment stones, which are distinguished based on morphological and physical-chemical criteria. Cholesterol stones are far more common (90% of all gallstones); in contrast to pigment stones, they contain more than 50% cholesterol by weight. The biochemical and metabolic pathways of cholesterol and bile synthesis are depicted in *figure 1*. The current hypothesis is that the primary pathophysiological defect in cholesterol stone formation is hepatic hypersecretion of cholesterol. Biliary cholesterol is solubilised by a complex mixture of lipid aggregates (mixed micelles and vesicles), composed of bile salts and phospholipids (mainly phosphatidylcholine = lecithin). If bile contains more cholesterol than can be solubilised by mixed micelles, crystals can precipitate, grow and agglomerate to form macroscopic stones. Furthermore, additional defects have been observed, including gallbladder hypomotility, gallbladder wall inflammation, mucin hypersecretion, and an imbalance of promoter- and inhibitor proteins, all of which contribute to gallstone formation [4].

Twin and family studies

Studies in mono- and dizygotic twins provide evidence for genetic factors in gallstone formation. In contrast to many early anecdotal reports of concordant monozygotic twins, which do not prove a causative role of genes, subsequent small unbiased **twin studies** confirmed the importance of genetic susceptibility. In one of the earliest studies, a preponderance of concordant pairs among monozygotic twins compared to dizygotic pairs of the same sex was found in 101 Danish twins with gallstones [5]. In an Australian series of twins, concordance was demonstrated in nine of 23 monozygotic twins but only in four out of 42 dizygotic pairs of the same sex [6]. Recently, these historical observations were confirmed by a large epidemiological study, which investigated 43,411 twins from the Swedish Twin Registry [7]. In this survey the concordance rate for gallstones was significantly higher in monozygotic compared to dizygotic twins (12% *vs* 6%) for both genders, and even higher differences were found in the younger twin cohorts. However, the rather low concordance rate of monozygotic twins also points to the importance of environmental factors and gene-environment interactions. Nevertheless, employing structural equation modelling (SEM), additive genetic effects were estimated to explain 25-41% of the total variance of the trait in the Swedish twin study [7].

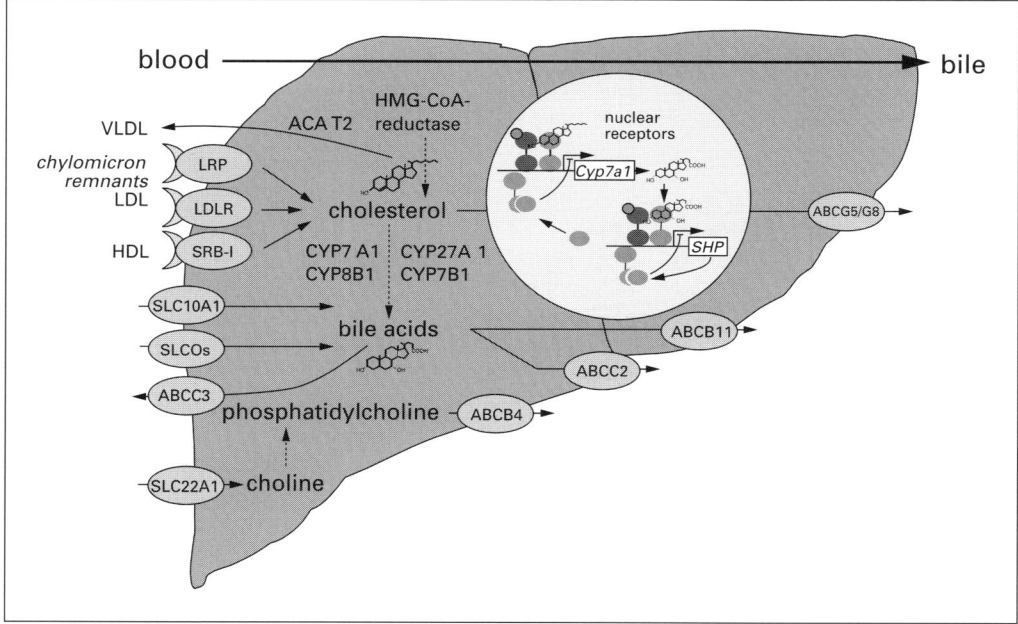

Figure 1. Schematic diagram of major pathways in hepatic cholesterol, bile salt and phosphatidylcholine (lecithin) metabolism. All genes involved in up-take, regulation of metabolism and secretion of cholesterol, bile salts and phosphatidylcholine into bile are potential candidates for cholesterol gallstone *("LITH")* genes. Until now only variations in the *ABCB4* gene encoding the hepatocanalicular phosphatidylcholine transporter have been unequivocally associated with gallstone disease. Abbreviations: ABC, ATP binding cassette transporter; ACAT, acyl-CoA cholesterol acyltransferase; CYP, cytochrome P450; HMG-CoA; 3-hydroxy-3-methylglutaryl coenzyme A; LDLR, LDL receptor; LRP, LDL receptor related protein; SHP, short heterodimer partner; SLC, solute carrier; SLCO, organic anion carrier; SR, scavenger receptor.

In a unique study of biliary lipid composition in twins, Kesäniemi *et al.* [8] randomly selected 35 male twin pairs from the Finnish Twin Cohort. Gallstones were ascertained by oral cholecystography or history of cholecystectomy in seven monozygotic (two concordant pairs) and three dizygotic patients (no concordant pair). The serum concentrations of methylsterols, which reflect hepatic cholesterol biosynthesis, the molar percentage of biliary cholesterol, and the biliary deoxycholate content as an index of bile lithogenicity [9] showed significant correlations in monozygotic but not dizygotic twins [8]. These observations support the hypothesis that biliary lipid composition as the major determinant of gallstone formation is also under significant genetic control.

The genetic background of gallstone formation is also illustrated by systematic **family studies**. Although several studies have documented that the gallstone prevalence is two to five times higher in first-degree relatives of stone patients [10], familial clustering of gallstones does not necessarily reflect genetic factors. Therefore van der Linden [11] studied the occurrence of gallstone disease in husbands and wives who had lived together continuously and had thus been exposed to the same environmental factors. In these investigations [11], the prevalence of symptomatic stones among women married to patients with gallstone diseases did not differ from that among women married to the patients' stone-free brothers, indicating that familial occurrence of gallstone disease is not primarily due to shared environmental but rather to genetic factors. Since genetic susceptibility should be particularly evident in parents of young gallstone patients, van der Linden [11] also demonstrated that the incidence in first-degree relatives of young gallstone carriers under 22 years differed significantly from those of age- and sex-matched controls.

Linkage studies in humans

An experimentally sophisticated approach for the assessment of genetic contribution to gallstone disease was recently presented by Duggirala *et al.* [12]. In this study variance component analysis (VCA) was employed in 32 Mexican-American families in order to systematically investigate the genetic determinants of symptomatic gallbladder disease. After adjustment for the significant effects of age, leptin, total cholesterol, and HDL cholesterol in males, heritability for gallbladder disease was high ($h^2 = 0.44 \pm 0.18$) and comparable to the heritability of type 2 diabetes mellitus and obesity [12]. These results have recently been confirmed in another American study [13]. Here, the additive genetic heritability of symptomatic gallbladder disease was 0.29 ± 0.14, as assessed by VCA with age and gender as significant co-variates [13].

In follow-up of the San Antonio Family Diabetes Study, Duggirala *et al.* [14] performed a genome-wide scan for gallstone susceptibility loci in 349 individuals, employing genetic markers at an average distance of 10 cM and multipoint VCA. Interestingly, a significant difference between the genetic susceptibility to symptomatic *versus* asymptomatic gallstone disease was noted; heritability was considerably high in patients with a history of cholecystectomy ($h^2 = 0.50$) but low if asymptomatic stone carriers (detected by ultrasound) were included in the analysis ($h^2 = 0.19$). In this study, significant genetic linkage (LOD scores 3.5-4.1) for symptomatic cholelithiasis was observed at the microsatellite marker *D11S1984* on human chromosome 11p [14]. A similar family-based genome-wide search for gallstone susceptibility loci in a Chinese population could identify suggestive linkage for three *"LITH"* loci on chromosomes 3, 9, and 11 [15].

In conclusion, both epidemiological and genetic linkage studies strongly suggest that genetic susceptibility plays a crucial role in gallstone pathogenesis. However, gallstone disease does not follow a simple (Mendelian) pattern of inheritance, but is a complex trait that is characterised by multiple interactions of various environmental and genetic risk factors. In order to further unravel the genetic basis for gallstone disease, animal studies and human association studies have been successfully employed [10, 16]. A combination of both approaches for the identification of susceptibility loci takes into account that the mammalian genome is highly conserved and that the same critical set of genes is rate-limiting in the pathogenesis of complex traits, such as gallstone formation [16]. As a result, risk loci identified in mice can subsequently be tested for association with the same trait in human studies *(figure 2, table I)*.

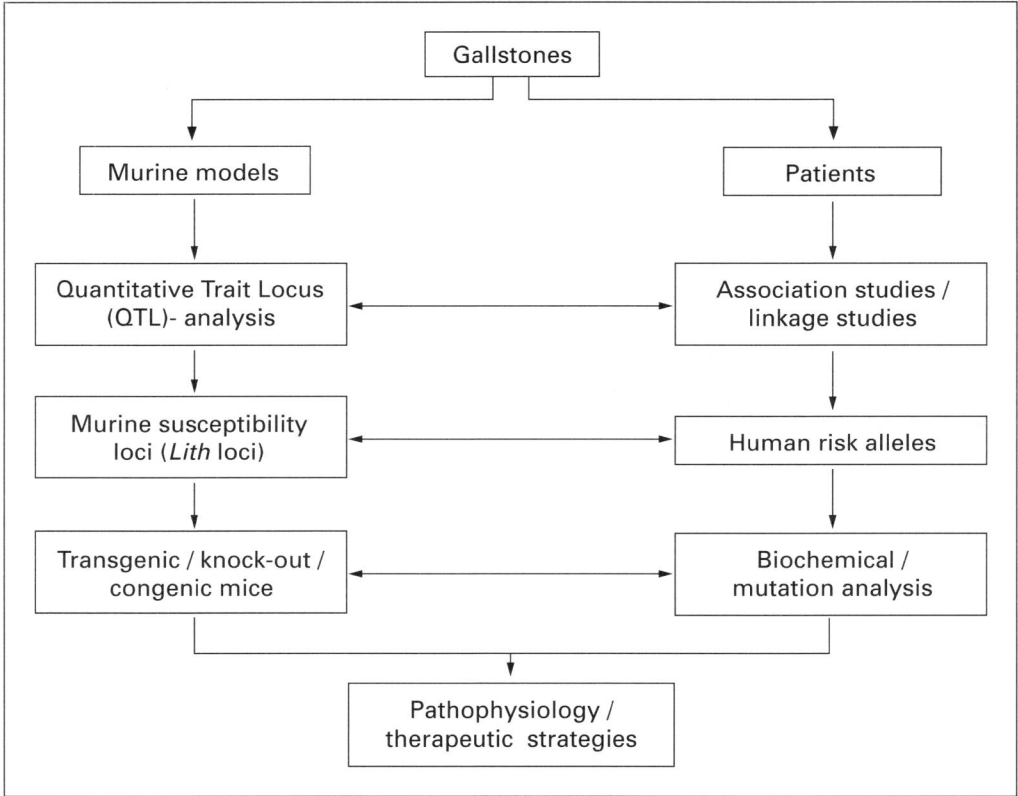

Figure 2. Schematic diagram of complementary research strategies for the identification of gallstone *("LITH")* genes.

Table I. Human association studies of candidate gallstone genes

Gene	Polymorphism	Population	Number of stone patients/controls	Allele frequencies stone patients: controls	Study
CYP7A1	5'-end variants	Mexican Americans	232/n.a.[a]	0.39: n.a.	[26]
APOE	ε4	Chile	110/109	0.10: 0.08	[36]
	ε4	Finland	169/200	0.16: 0.20	[35]
	ε2	Finland	148/896	0.02: 0.04*	[34]
	ε4	Germany	184/184	0.13: 0.13	[46]
	ε4	Japan	79/53	0.08: 0.09	[37]
	ε4	Netherlands	31/21[b]	0.26: 0.14*	[40, 41]
	ε4	Spain	221/125	0.11: 0.04**	[33]
APOB	XbaI RFLP	Finland	91/92	0.42: 0.39	[44]
		China	190/441	0.11: 0.04**	[42]
CETP	TaqIB RFLP	Finland	91/92	0.51: 0.40*	[44]
		Germany	184/184	0.39: 0.42	[46]
LDLR	(dTA)$_n$	China	131	0.40: 0.27*	[49]

[a] n.a., not available.
[b] Recurrence after ESWL/no recurrence.
* $P < 0.05$; ** $P < 0.01$, stone patients vs controls.
Abbreviations: APO, apolipoprotein; CETP, cholesteryl ester transfer protein; CYP, cytochrome P45; LDLR, low density lipoprotein receptor; RFLP, restriction fragment length polymorphism.

Gallstone genes

ABC transporter B4 *(ABCB4)*

In 2001, the first report about a single gene defect causing gallstone formation in a defined subgroup of individuals, *i.e.* young patients with a symptomatic and recurring form of cholelithiasis, was published [17]. In the study by Rosmorduc *et al.* [17], six patients with this 'peculiar' form of gallstone disease were investigated. In two of these patients, physical-chemical analysis showed a marked supersaturation of hepatic bile with cholesterol together with low phospholipid concentrations. Based on these observations, the disorder was named *"Low Phospholipid-Associated Cholelithiasis"* (LPAC syndrome) [17]. Phosphatidylcholine is primarily transported into bile by the hepatocanalicular transporter ABCB4 *(figure 1)*, formerly known as MDR3 (Multidrug Resistance P-glycoprotein 3). Therefore, these observations led to a systematic search for mutations in the corresponding *ABCB4* gene. Heterozygous and homozygous *ABCB4* gene point mutations were identified in 18 out of 32 patients (56%), who presented with the clinical characteristics of the LPAC syndrome *(table II)*, whereas no *ABCB4* mutations were found in 28 patients with "classic" gallstone disease and 33 without a history of cholelithiasis [18]. Importantly, the pathophysiological basis for the human LPAC syndrome is consistent with the spontaneous occurrence of cholecysto- and hepatolithiasis in knockout mice with biliary phosphatidylcholine deficiency due to disruption of the orthologous mouse *Abcb4* gene [19]. In these mice, needle-shaped cholesterol crystals and stones are observed in a progressive age-dependent fashion. Of note, intrahepatic duct stones are observed in female knockout mice after the development of fibro-obliteration and segmental strictures in bile ducts [20]. Thus, the $Abcb4^{-/-}$ mouse model also resembles primary sclerosing cholangitis and chronic idiopathic cholangitis.

Table II. Clinical and genetic characteristics of *"Low Phospholipid-Associated Cholelithiasis"* (LPAC syndrome)

- Age at onset of symptoms < 40 years
- Cholesterol gallbladder stones and intrahepatic sludge or microlithiasis (hyperechoic foci upon ultrasound examination)
- Recurrence of biliary symptoms after cholecystectomy
- Positive family history
- Mild chronic cholestasis
- 33% Association with intrahepatic cholestasis of pregnancy
- 56% *ABCB4* mutations
- Prevention by hydrophilic bile acids

Comparable to the animal model, homozygous *ABCB4* mutations that lead to complete absence of the ABCB4 protein and virtually no secretion of phosphatidylcholine into bile result in progressive familial intrahepatic cholestasis (type 3) and early liver cirrhosis in childhood [21]. In the latter study [21], *ABCB4* mutations were detected in 54% of patients with progressive familiar intrahepatic cholestasis type 3. Of note, gallbladder stones were also observed in a number a patients. Furthermore, low hepatic expression levels of ABCB4 and phosphatidylcholine transfer protein occur together with markedly reduced biliary phosphatidylcholine concentrations in Asian patients with primary cholesterol hepatolithiasis [22].

The results of the French studies [17, 18] are also reinforced by a study that demonstrated biliary phospholipid deficiency in patients with cholesterol microlithiasis [23] and a case report which identified an *ABCB4* mutation in a patient who presented with cholelithiasis in adolescence, followed by recurrent intrahepatic cholestasis of pregnancy and finally biliary cirrhosis in adulthood [24]. Taken together these studies demonstrate that *ABCB4* gene mutations represent an important risk factor for specific forms of cholelithiasis.

In contrast to *ABCB4*, no associations between gallstone formation and the genes encoding the hepatocanalicular transporters for cholesterol *(ABCG5/G8)* and bile salts *(ABCB11)* have yet been established. Genetic variants of these transporters are expected to contribute to cholesterol hypersecretion and bile salt hyposecretion, and early-onset cholesterol cholelithiasis or benign recurrent familial intrahepatic cholestasis could represent defined clinical subgroups that might be linked to specific mutations in *ABCB5/G8* and *ABCB11*, respectively.

Cholesterol 7α-hydroxylase *(CYP7A1)*

CYP7A1 is an attractive candidate gene because it encodes the rate-limiting enzyme in the classic pathway for hepatic bile salt synthesis. As described, bile salts are essential for keeping cholesterol molecules solubilised in mixed micelles in bile. Patients with homozygous *CYPA1* mutations display hypertriglyceridemia and hypercholesterolemia resistant to HMG-CoA reductase inhibitors, whereas fecal bile salt excretion is markedly deficient [25]. Clinically important, gallstone formation has been reported in two brothers who underwent cholecystectomy for gallstones at age 40 to 42 [25]. A common link between *CYP7A1* and the appearance of gallstones is supported by a case-control study in 232 Mexican-Americans. In this investigation, a variant allele of the 5' end of the gene was detected twice as often in patients compared to controls and was significantly associated with gallstones in men (but not in women) [26]. Additional evidence for the importance of *CYP7A1* in gallstone pathogenesis has been provided by mouse genetics. When fed an atherogenic diet, non-transgenic littermates, but not *Cyp7a1* overexpressing transgenic mice, accumulate cholesterol and cholesterol esters in their livers and plasma. The ability of *Cyp7a1* transgenic mice to maintain cholesterol and lipoprotein homeostasis completely prevented the formation of gallstones (and atherosclerosis) in these animals [27]. However, in contrast to rodents, human *CYP7A1* is not induced by dietary cholesterol. *Cyp7a1* knockout mice over-expressing human *CYP7A1* regulate bile salt pool size and plasma cholesterol levels independently of CYP7A1 activity, thus challenging the concept of CYP7A1 as the main determinant of plasma cholesterol regulation [28].

Apolipoprotein E (ApoE)

The most extensively studied gene variants in gallstone patients are apolipoprotein E polymorphisms [29]. ApoE is the major protein component of triglyceride-rich lipoproteins (VLDL, LDL) and serves as the high-affinity ligand for the hepatic LDL receptor and the LDL receptor-related protein. Overall, three main codominant *APOE* alleles (ε2, ε3, ε4) exist, which lead to arginine to cysteine substitutions at amino acid positions 112 and/or 158 and result in six different ApoE isoforms (E2/E2, E3/E3, E4/E4, E2/E3, E2/E4, E3/E4). These amino acid substitutions cause differences in receptor-binding affinities and catabolic rates of the isoforms, thus determining serum levels and clearance rates of circulating lipoproteins [30]. Individuals carrying the E2/E2 isoform have 11-14 mg/dl lower serum (LDL) cholesterol concentrations as compared to persons with the E3/E3 isoform; compared to the latter isoform, subjects carrying the ε4 allele in homozygous or heterozygous state display even higher serum cholesterol levels [31].

In recent studies, the presence of the ε4 allele has been associated with coronary heart disease and Alzheimer disease [32]. The ε4 allele has also been associated with cholelithasis in a carefully designed case-control study [33]. The ε4 allele frequency was shown to be significantly higher in 221 symptomatic and asymptomatic patients with gallstone disease compared to in-hospital controls with other gastroenterological disorders. Contrary, the ApoE2 isoform has been shown to be inversely correlated to gallstone disease [34]. ApoE2 was found less frequently in women with gallstone disease compared to women with gallstones (OR 0.28, 95% CI 0.08-0.92); interestingly, this protective effect of ApoE2 was not evident in males, but was independent of known risk factors for gallstone disease like diabetes, elevated serum triglycerides and insulin levels in women [34].

Albeit the association between ApoE isoforms and gallstone disease was not found in three other case-control studies [35-37], the latter studies might have been biased by inclusion of younger control patients [29]. Taken together the ApoE association studies demonstrate an overall difference of 15-25% with respect to the presence of the ε4 allele in homozygous or heterozygous state between gallstone patients and controls. Furthermore, a knockout mouse model supports the relevance of ApoE for stone formation. When *Apoe* knockout mice are fed a high-cholesterol or lithogenic diet, the increases of biliary cholesterol secretion and cholesterol saturation are lower compared to wild-type mice [38, 39], and gallstone formation is augmented [38]. In addition, a Dutch study was able to show a significantly higher recurrence rate of gallstones after extracorporeal shock wave lithotripsy (ESWL) in subjects carrying the ε4 allele [40, 41].

Apolipoprotein B (ApoB)

ApoB is the only apolipoprotein of LDL and functions as a ligand for receptor-mediated endocytosis of LDL, which is a major determinant of hepatic cholesterol uptake and serum cholesterol levels. Several *APOB* gene polymorphisms have been associated with differences in serum cholesterol concentrations and complex disorders like coronary heart disease and type 2 diabetes mellitus. A significant association between the X+ allele of a common restriction fragment length polymorphism (RFLP) in exon 26 (XbaI) and cholesterol gallstone prevalence as well as increased total cholesterol, LDL cholesterol and ApoB concentrations in serum has been detected in a Chinese case-control study [42]. Although the lipid profile in the latter study is not representative for stone patients in Europe [10], the genetic association might be related to decreased LDL receptor affinity for ApoB. In line with the latter study, heterozygosity (*APOB* X+/X-) has also been reported to be associated with gallstone disease (and gallbladder cancer) in India [43]. In contrast, in an earlier study from Finland the frequency of X+ alleles did not differ between stone patients and controls, but was significantly higher in patients with cholesterolosis compared to those with cholesterol gallstones [44].

Cholesteryl ester transfer protein *(CETP)*

CETP has been shown to play an important role in the catabolism of HDL cholesteryl esters and reverse cholesterol transport from peripheral organs to the liver in humans. CETP facilitates the exchange of neutral lipids among plasma lipoproteins and transfers cholesteryl esters from HDL to triglyceride-rich lipoproteins (VLDL, LDL) in exchange for triglycerides. Whereas CETP is absent in mice, the importance of CETP was demonstrated in a recent study showing that the CETP inhibitor torcetrapib markedly increased HDL cholesterol levels in patients with low HDL [45]. In contrast, humans with high CETP activity display low HDL cholesterol as well as high VLDL triglyceride levels, a pattern of plasma lipids that is associated with an increased risk of gallstones [10]. In a Finish study, a TaqIB RFLP of the gene encoding the cholesteryl ester transfer protein was shown to be associated with both serum HDL cholesterol levels and cholesterol stones [44]. Although we were not able to confirm the association between this polymorphism and the presence of gallstones in German patients, HDL concentrations were associated with TaqIB genotypes in females [46], consistent with previous reports [47, 48].

LDL receptor gene family

A dinucleotide repeat polymorphism at the 3'-end of the LDL receptor *(LDLR)* gene has been shown to be associated with cholesterol gallstone disease in a study from China [49]. The multiligand receptor Megalin, another member of the LDLR gene family also known as LDLR-related protein 2, is not expressed in hepatocytes but on the apical surfaces of specialised epithelia. These include the proximal renal tubules and the distal small intestine, where Megalin mediates the endocytotic uptake of vitamins A and D_3, and vitamin B_{12}, respectively [50]. Interestingly, the Megalin gene co-localizes (together with the bile salt export pump) in the refined gallstone susceptibility locus *Lith1* on chromosome 2 of the murine genetic "gallstone map" [16]. Two Megalin single nucleotide polymorphisms (SNPs) have been reported to be associated with the presence of cholecystolithiasis and serum HDL cholesterol levels in Caucasian patients [46]. These findings point to a potential role of Megalin, which also binds ApoE-containing lipoproteins, in HDL cholesterol metabolism and/or epithelial cell function during gallstone pathogenesis.

Cholecystokinin A receptor *(CCKAR)*

Beside the genes involved in hepatic cholesterol metabolism, genes governing gallbladder function might participate in the pathogenesis of gallstone disease. Stasis of supersaturated bile in the gallbladder favours cholesterol crystallization and gallstone formation. Furthermore, a number of studies have documented increased fasting and postprandial volumes in gallstone patients [10]. A hormone clearly related to gallbladder motility is cholecystokinin. It is synthesised in specialised proximal small intestinal crypt cells, released postprandially by fatty and amino acids, and induces profound gallbladder contraction. Altered CCKAR primary structure has been associated with gallstone formation in a subgroup of gallstone patients [51]. In a single obese patient with cholesterol gallstone disease, Miller *et al.* [52] found abnormal processing of the *CCKAR* mRNA, which yielded transcripts without exon 3 and resulted in a non-functional receptor. Although further screening did not detect any mutations in the coding region of the *CCKAR* gene in gallstone patients [53-55], a potential pathophysiological link between *CCKAR* and gallstone formation is supported by knockout mice with homozygous disruption of the orthologous mouse *Cckar* gene. These mice display profound gallbladder hypomotility and form significantly more gallstones than wild-type mice [53, 56]. As inferred from increased cholesterol absorption efficiency, they may also exhibit prolonged intestinal transit time, as has been shown for human gallstone patients [57].

In addition to *CCKAR*, gene variants of other receptors and transmembrane signal transducers expressed by gallbladder epithelia might also contribute to gallbladder hypomotility and predispose to gallstones. Recently gene polymorphisms that result in amino acid substitutions within the α_3-adrenergic receptor *(ADRB3)* and the G-protein-β_3-subunit *(GNB3)* were observed more frequently in female or lean gallstone patients, respectively, albeit overall allele frequencies did not differ from (historical) controls [58, 59].

Cystic fibrosis transmembrane conductance regulator (CFTR) / ABC transporter C7 (ABCC7)

Cystic fibrosis (CF) is caused by mutations in the *ABCC7* gene that encodes the CF transmembrane conductance regulator (CFTR), a cAMP-dependent Cl⁻ channel. The gallstone prevalence in CF is at least 10-30% compared with less than 5% in age-matched controls. In contrast to earlier studies [60], Angelico et al. [61] found no significant changes in cholesterol saturation between patients with cystic fibrosis with and without gallstones, and gallstones from CF patients were "black" pigment stones composed mainly of polymerised calcium bilirubinate and protein, whereas their cholesterol contents were 28-44% only. Consistent with the human phenotype, CF mouse models display bile salt malabsorption, elevated bilirubin secretion rates ("hyperbilirubinbilia"), hepatic deposition of calcium and iron most likely as monoacid bilirubinates, and a high gallstone prevalence [62].

Ileal bile salt transporter (SLC10A2)

The ileal sodium-coupled bile salt transporter (official gene name "Solute Carrier 10A2") reabsorbs bile salt conjugates in the distal small intestine [63]. Point mutations in *SLC10A2* can lead to primary bile salt malabsorption with concomitant chronic diarrhoea, failure to thrive, and reduced plasma levels of cholesterol and fat soluble vitamins [64]. "Milder" defects may lead to bile salt "spillage" into the colon, a prerequisite for intestinal absorption and subsequent enterohepatic cycling of unconjugated bilirubin, which increases bilirubin levels in bile ("hyperbilirubinbilia") [65]. The monoacid salt of calcium bilirubinate is invariably found in small amounts in the cores of "cholesterol" stones [10], indicating that bilirubinate might play a role in the earliest events of cholesterol nucleation. However, *SLC10A2* does not appear to be a candidate gene for cholesterol gallstone formation, but might be implicated in the formation of "black" pigment gallstones. Recently one patient with pigment stones was reported who carries a heterozygous missense mutation that abolishes taurocholate transport activity and decreases SLC10A2 expression *in vitro* [66]. This observation is consistent with the hypothesis that a subgroup of patients develops pigment stones due to bile salt malabsorption caused by SLC10A2 deficiency.

Conclusions

The identification of new gallstone genes is based on two experimental approaches *(figure 2)*. Firstly, important information on gallstone genes can be derived from animal studies, in particular crossbreeding experiments in inbred mouse strains that differ in genetic susceptibility to gallstone formation (quantitative trait locus [QTL] analysis) [16, 67, 68]. Employing this technique, numerous candidate genes for cholesterol gallstone susceptibility have already been identified in the mouse genome [16]. These include the hepatocanalicular transporters for biliary lipids *(ABCB11, ABCG5/G8, ABCC2)*, the nuclear receptors that regulate these genes (FXR, LXRα, PPARγ), and biliary mucins [16, 67, 69, 70].

The second, complementary approach for the identification of new candidate gallstone genes is based on human association studies. A widely used and successful method to establish genetic factors for complex traits is the case-control design *(table I)*. However, case-control studies have certain limitations, including the preponderance of clinically diagnosed cases, which might represent the more severe end of the disease spectrum, potentially biased control groups, low statistical power due to small sample sizes, and linkage disequilibrium between gene polymorphisms [71, 72]. The latter difficulties can, at least in part, be circumvented by the use of haplotype analysis [73]. Haplotypes are defined as characteristic combinations of polymorphisms on single chromosomes and can be reconstructed from genotype data in population samples using novel algorithms [74]. In complex diseases, haplotype analysis might provide more information than analysis of individual gene polymorphisms, and due to the reduced statistical power a genotype-phenotype association can even be missed if only single polymorphisms are investigated instead of haplotypes [75]. This new experimental approach for the identification of gallstone genes will greatly benefit from the further delineation of the complete haplotype map of the human genome [76].

In summary, the combination of complementary genetic strategies in mice and humans, together with further pathophysiological studies of gallstone disease will guide the identification of novel preventive and therapeutic strategies for this exceptionally prevalent disease.

Acknowledgements : Experimental work of the authors related to the molecular genetics of cholesterol gallstone formation has been supported in part by research grants from *Deutsche Forschungsgemeinschaft* (LA997/3-1) and *Ministerium für Wissenschaft und Forschung des Landes Nordrhein-Westfalen* (to F.L.).

References

1. Carey MC, Paigen B. Epidemiology of the American Indians' burden and its likely genetic origins. *Hepatology* 2002; 36: 781-91.
2. Brett M, Barker DJ. The world distribution of gallstones. *Int J Epidemiol* 1976; 5: 335-41.
3. Kratzer W, Mason RA, Kachele V. Prevalence of gallstones in sonographic surveys worldwide. *J Clin Ultrasound* 1999; 27: 1-7.
4. Kosters A, Jirsa M, Groen AK. Genetic background of cholesterol gallstone disease. *Biochim Biophys Acta* 2003; 1637: 1-19.
5. Harvald B, Hauge M. A catamnestic investigation of Danish twins. A preliminary report. *Dan Med Bull* 1956; 3: 150-8.
6. Doig RK. Illness in twins. III. Cholelithiasis. *Med J Aust* 1957; 44: 716-7.
7. Katsika D, Grjibovski A, Lammert F, Einarsson C, Lichtenstein P, Marschall HU. Genetic and environmental influences for gallstone-related diagnoses: a Swedish twin study of 43,141 twin pairs. *J Hepatol* 2004; 40 (Suppl. 1): 4A.
8. Kesäniemi YA, Koskenvuo M, Vuoristo M, Miettinen TA. Biliary lipid composition in monozygotic and dizygotic pairs of twins. *Gut* 1989; 30: 1750-6.
9. Figge A, Lammert F, Paigen B, Henkel A, Matern S, Korstanje R, Shneider BL, *et al*. Hepatic overexpression of murine Abcb11 increases hepatobiliary lipid secretion and reduces hepatic steatosis. *J Biol Chem* 2004; 279: 2790-9.

10. Paigen B, Carey MC. Gallstones. In: King RA, Rotter JF, Motulsky AG, eds. *The genetic basis of common diseases*. London: Oxford University Press, 2002: 298-335.
11. Van der Linden W. Genetic factors in gallstone disease. *Clin Gastroenterol* 1973; 2: 603-14.
12. Duggirala R, Mitchell BD, Blangero J, Stern MP. Genetic determinants of variation in gallbladder disease in the Mexican-American population. *Genet Epidemiol* 1999; 16: 191-204.
13. Nakeeb A, Comuzzie AG, Martin L, Sonnenberg GE, Swartz-Basile D, Kissebah AH, Pitt HA. Gallstones: genetics *versus* environment. *Ann Surg* 2002; 235: 842-9.
14. Duggirala R, Dodd GD, Fowler S, Schneider J, Arya R, Diehl AK, Almasy L, et al. A major susceptibility locus for gallbladder disease is on chromosome 11p in Mexican Americans. *Am J Hum Genet* 2003; 73: A167.
15. Han T, Yuan W, Qin J, Fei J, Jiang Z, Jin L, Zhang S, et al. A genomewide scan for the susceptibility loci to cholelithiasis in Chinese population. *Am J Hum Genet* 2003; 73: A1929.
16. Lammert F, Carey MC, Paigen B. Chromosomal organization of candidate genes involved in cholesterol gallstone formation: a murine gallstone map. *Gastroenterology* 2001; 120: 221-38.
17. Rosmorduc O, Hermelin B, Poupon R. MDR3 gene defect in adults with symptomatic intrahepatic and gallbladder cholesterol cholelithiasis. *Gastroenterology* 2001; 120: 1459-67.
18. Rosmorduc O, Hermelin B, Boelle PY, Parc R, Taboury J, Poupon R. ABCB4 gene mutation-associated cholelithiasis in adults. *Gastroenterology* 2003; 125: 452-9.
19. Lammert F, Wang DQ, Hillebrandt S, Geier A, Fickert P, Trauner M, Matern S, et al. Spontaneous cholecysto- and hepatolithiasis in *Mdr2-/-* mice: a model for low phospholipid-associated cholelithiasis. *Hepatology* 2004; 39: 117-28.
20. Fickert P, Zollner G, Fuchsbichler A, Stumptner C, Weiglein AH, Lammert F, Marschall HU, Tsybrovskyy O, Zatloukal K, Denk H, Trauner M. Ursodeoxycholic acid aggravates bile infarcts in bile duct-ligated and *Mdr2* knockout mice via disruption of cholangioles. *Gastroenterology* 2002; 123: 1238-51.
21. Jacquemin E, de Vree JM, Cresteil D, Sokal EM, Sturm E, Dumont M, Scheffer GL, et al. The wide spectrum of multidrug resistance 3 deficiency: from neonatal cholestasis to cirrhosis of adulthood. *Gastroenterology* 2001; 120: 1448-58.
22. Shoda J, Oda K, Suzuki H, Sugiyama Y, Ito K, Cohen DE, Feng L, et al. Etiologic significance of defects in cholesterol, phospholipid, and bile acid metabolism in the liver of patients with intrahepatic calculi. *Hepatology* 2001; 33: 1194-205.
23. Fracchia M, Pellegrino S, Secreto P, Gallo L, Masoero G, Pera A, Galatola G. Biliary lipid composition in cholesterol microlithiasis. *Gut* 2001; 48: 702-6.
24. Lucena JF, Herrero JI, Quiroga J, Sangro B, Garcia-Foncillas J, Zabalegui N, Sola J, et al. A multidrug resistance 3 gene mutation causing cholelithiasis, cholestasis of pregnancy, and adulthood biliary cirrhosis. *Gastroenterology* 2003; 124: 1037-42.
25. Pullinger CR, Eng C, Salen G, Shefer S, Batta AK, Erickson SK, Verhagen A, et al. Human cholesterol 7α-hydroxylase (CYP7A1) deficiency has a hypercholesterolemic phenotype. *J Clin Invest* 2002; 110: 109-17.
26. Lin JP, Hanis CL, Boerwinkle E. Genetic epidemiology of gallbladder disease in Mexican-Americans and cholesterol 7α-hydroxylase gene variation. *Am J Hum Genet* 1994; 55: A48.
27. Miyake JH, Duong-Polk XT, Taylor JM, Du EZ, Castellani LW, Lusis AJ, Davis RA. Transgenic expression of cholesterol 7α-hydroxylase prevents atherosclerosis in C57BL/6J mice. *Arterioscler Thromb Vasc Biol* 2002; 22: 121-6.
28. Tiemann M, Han Z, Soccio R, Bollineni J, Shefer S, Sehayek E, Breslow JL. Cholesterol feeding of mice expressing cholesterol 7α-hydroxylase increases bile acid pool size despite decreased enzyme activity. *Proc Natl Acad Sci USA* 2004; 101: 1846-51.
29. Van Erpecum KJ, Carey MC. Apolipoprotein E4: another risk factor for cholesterol gallstone formation? *Gastroenterology* 1996; 111: 1764-7.

30. Mahley RW. Apolipoprotein E: cholesterol transport protein with expanding role in cell biology. *Science* 1988; 240: 622-30.
31. Sing CF, Davignon J. Role of the apolipoprotein E polymorphism in determining normal plasma lipid and lipoprotein variation. *Am J Hum Genet* 1985; 37: 268-85.
32. Eichner JE, Dunn ST, Perveen G, Thompson DM, Stewart KE, Stroehla BC. Apolipoprotein E polymorphism and cardiovascular disease: a HuGE review. *Am J Epidemiol* 2002; 155: 487-95.
33. Bertomeu A, Ros E, Zambon D, Vela M, Perez-Ayuso RM, Targarona E, Trias M, et al. Apolipoprotein E polymorphism and gallstones. *Gastroenterology* 1996; 111: 1603-10.
34. Niemi M, Kervinen K, Rantala A, Kauma H, Paivansalo M, Savolainen MJ, Lilja M, et al. The role of apolipoprotein E and glucose intolerance in gallstone disease in middle aged subjects. *Gut* 1999; 44: 557-62.
35. Juvonen T, Kervinen K, Kairaluoma MI, Lajunen LH, Kesaniemi YA. Gallstone cholesterol content is related to apolipoprotein E polymorphism. *Gastroenterology* 1993; 104: 1806-13.
36. Rollan A, Loyola G, Covarrubias C, Giancaspero R, Acevedo K, Nervi F. Apolipoprotein E polymorphism in patients with acute pancreatitis. *Pancreas* 1994; 9: 349-53.
37. Hasegawa K, Terada S, Kubota K, Itakura H, Imamura H, Ohnishi S, Aoki T, et al. Effect of apolipoprotein E polymorphism on bile lipid composition and the formation of cholesterol gallstone. *Am J Gastroenterol* 2003; 98: 1605-9.
38. Amigo L, Quinones V, Mardones P, Zanlungo S, Miquel JF, Nervi F, Rigotti A. Impaired biliary cholesterol secretion and decreased gallstone formation in apolipoprotein E-deficient mice fed a high-cholesterol diet. *Gastroenterology* 2000; 118: 772-9.
39. Sehayek E, Shefer S, Nguyen LB, Ono JG, Merkel M, Breslow JL. Apolipoprotein E regulates dietary cholesterol absorption and biliary cholesterol excretion: studies in C57BL/6 apolipoprotein E knockout mice. *Proc Natl Acad Sci USA* 2000; 97: 3433-7.
40. Portincasa P, van Erpecum KJ, van De Meeberg PC, Dallinga-Thie GM, de Bruin TW, van Berge-Henegouwen GP. Apolipoprotein E4 genotype and gallbladder motility influence speed of gallstone clearance and risk of recurrence after extracorporeal shock-wave lithotripsy. *Hepatology* 1996; 24: 580-7.
41. Venneman NG, van Berge-Henegouwen GP, Portincasa P, Stolk MF, Vos A, Plaisier PW, van Erpecum KJ. Absence of apolipoprotein E4 genotype, good gallbladder motility and presence of solitary stones delay rather than prevent gallstone recurrence after extracorporeal shock wave lithotripsy. *J Hepatol* 2001; 35: 10-6.
42. Han T, Jiang Z, Suo G, Zhang S. Apolipoprotein B-100 gene XbaI polymorphism and cholesterol gallstone disease. *Clin Genet* 2000; 57: 304-8.
43. Mittal B, Mittal RD. Genetics of gallstone disease. *J Postgrad Med* 2002; 48: 149-52.
44. Juvonen T, Savolainen MJ, Kairaluoma MI, Lajunen LH, Humphries SE, Kesaniemi YA. Polymorphisms at the apoB, apoA-I, and cholesteryl ester transfer protein gene loci in patients with gallbladder disease. *J Lipid Res* 1995; 36: 804-12.
45. Brousseau ME, Schaefer EJ, Wolfe ML, Bloedon LT, Digenio AG, Clark RW, Mancuso JP, Rader DJ. Effects of an inhibitor of cholesteryl ester transfer protein on HDL cholesterol. *N Engl J Med* 2004; 350: 1505-15.
46. Schirin-Sokhan R, Matern S, Lammert F. Human *LITH* genes: the gene encoding the multiligand receptor LRP2 is associated with cholecystolithiasis. *Hepatology* 2002; 36: 342A.
47. Ordovas JM, Cupples LA, Corella D, Otvos JD, Osgood D, Martinez A, Lahoz C, et al. Association of cholesteryl ester transfer protein-TaqIB polymorphism with variations in lipoprotein subclasses and coronary heart disease risk: the Framingham study. *Arterioscler Thromb Vasc Biol* 2000; 20: 1323-9.
48. Brousseau ME, O'Connor JJ, Ordovas JM, Collins D, Otvos JD, Massov T, McNamara JR, et al. Cholesteryl ester transfer protein TaqI B2B2 genotype is associated with higher HDL cholesterol levels and lower risk of coronary artery disease end points in men with HDL deficiency. *Arterioscler Thromb Vasc Biol* 2002; 22: 1148-54.

49. Feng D, Han T, Chen S. Polymorphism at the LDL receptor gene locus in patients with cholesterol gallstone disease. *Zhonghua Yi Xue Za Zhi* 1998; 78: 63-5.
50. Willnow TE, Nykjaer A, Herz J. Lipoprotein receptors: new roles for ancient proteins. *Nature Cell Biol* 1999; 1: E157-62.
51. Schneider H, Sanger P, Hanisch E. *In vitro* effects of cholecystokinin fragments on human gallbladders. Evidence for an altered CCK-receptor structure in a subgroup of patients with gallstones. *J Hepatol* 1997; 26: 1063-8.
52. Miller LJ, Holicky EL, Ulrich CD, Wieben ED. Abnormal processing of the human cholecystokinin receptor gene in association with gallstones and obesity. *Gastroenterology* 1995; 109: 1375-80.
53. Miyasaka K, Takata Y, Funakoshi A. Association of cholecystokinin A receptor gene polymorphism with cholelithiasis and the molecular mechanisms of this polymorphism. *J Gastroenterol* 2002; 37: S102-6.
54. Nardone G, Ferber IA, Miller LJ. The integrity of the cholecystokinin receptor gene in gallbladder disease and obesity. *Hepatology* 1995; 22: 1751-3.
55. Klass DM. Gene polymorphisms and impaired gallbladder motility. In: Adler G, Blum HE, Fuchs M, Stange EF, eds. *Falk Symposium 139. Gallstones: pathogenesis and treatment*. Freiburg, 2004; 35-6.
56. Schmitz F, Wang DQ, Blaeker M, Nguyen M, Chiu M, Beinborn M, Carey MC, et al. CCK-A receptor deficient mice have an increased susceptibility to cholesterol gallstones. *Hepatology* 1996; 24: 246A.
57. Shoda J, He BF, Tanaka N, Matsuzaki Y, Osuga T, Yamamori S, Miyazaki H, et al. Increase of deoxycholate in supersaturated bile of patients with cholesterol gallstone disease and its correlation with de novo syntheses of cholesterol and bile acids in liver, gallbladder emptying, and small intestinal transit. *Hepatology* 1995; 21: 1291-302.
58. Klass DM, Seneshaw M, Kratzer W, Adler G, Fuchs M. The G-protein-β-polypeptide 3 (GNB3 C825T) polymorphism is a risk factor for gallstone disease in lean subjects. In: Adler G, Blum HE, Fuchs M, Stange EF, eds. *Falk Symposium 139. Gallstones: pathogenesis and treatment*. Freiburg, 2004; A16.
59. Seneshaw M, Klass DM, Kratzer W, Adler G, Fuchs M. Heterozygosity for the b3-adrenergic receptor (Trp64Arg): a genetic marker for gallstone formation in women? In: Adler G, Blum HE, Fuchs M, Stange EF, eds. *Falk Symposium 139. Gallstones: pathogenesis and treatment*. Freiburg, 2004; A26.
60. Roy CC, Weber AM, Morin CL, Combes JC, Nussle D, Megevand A, Lasalle R. Abnormal biliary lipid composition in cystic fibrosis. Effect of pancreatic enzymes. *N Engl J Med* 1977; 297: 1301-5.
61. Angelico M, Gandin C, Canuzzi P, Bertasi S, Cantafora A, De Santis A, Quattrucci S, et al. Gallstones in cystic fibrosis: a critical reappraisal. *Hepatology* 1991; 14: 768-75.
62. Broderick AL, Hofmann AF, Carey MC. Correcting biliary phenotype in cystic fibrosis (CF) mice: nor-ursodeoxycholic acid (nor-UDCA), but not UDCA, normalizes hepatic bile pH and increases bile flow in G551D CF mice. *Hepatology* 2002; 36: A337.
63. Dawson PA. Intestinal bile acid transport: molecules, mechanisms, and malabsorption. In: Paumgartner G, Stiehl A, Gerok W, Keppler D, Leuschner U, eds. *Bile acids and cholestasis*. Dordrecht: Kluwer Academic Publishers, 1999; 1-28.
64. Oelkers P, Kirby LC, Heubi JE, Dawson PA. Primary bile acid malabsorption caused by mutations in the ileal sodium-dependent bile acid transporter gene (SLC10A2). *J Clin Invest* 1997; 99: 1880-7.
65. Brink MA, Slors JF, Keulemans YC, Mok KS, de Waart DR, Carey MC, Groen AK, et al. Enterohepatic cycling of bilirubin: a putative mechanism for pigment gallstone formation in ileal Crohn's disease. *Gastroenterology* 1999; 116: 1420-7.
66. Dawson PA, Montagnani M, Fusegawa H, Clarke G, Carey MC. Identification of a dysfunctional ileal bile acid transporter gene in a patient with pigment gallstones. *Hepatology* 2000; 32: 434A.

67. Lammert F, Wang DQ, Wittenburg H, Bouchard G, Hillebrandt S, Taenzler B, Carey MC, et al. *Lith* genes control mucin accumulation, cholesterol crystallization, and gallstone formation in A/J and AKR/J inbred mice. *Hepatology* 2002; 36: 1145-54.
68. Wittenburg H, Lyons MA, Paigen B, Carey MC. Mapping cholesterol gallstone susceptibility *(Lith)* genes in inbred mice. *Dig Liver Dis* 2003; 35 (Suppl. 3): S2-7.
69. Wittenburg H, Lyons MA, Li R, Churchill GA, Carey MC, Paigen B. FXR and ABCG5/ABCG8 as determinants of cholesterol gallstone formation from quantitative trait locus mapping in mice. *Gastroenterology* 2003; 125: 868-81.
70. Lyons MA, Wittenburg H, Li R, Walsh KA, Leonard MR, Korstanje R, Churchill GA, et al. *Lith6*: a new QTL for cholesterol gallstones from an intercross of CAST/Ei and DBA/2J inbred mouse strains. *J Lipid Res* 2003; 44: 1763-71.
71. Schulz KF, Grimes DA. Case-control studies: research in reverse. *Lancet* 2002; 359: 431-4.
72. Zondervan KT, Cardon LR. The complex interplay among factors that influence allelic association. *Nature Rev Genet* 2004; 5: 89-100.
73. Wasmuth HE, Matern S, Lammert F. From genotypes to haplotypes in hepatobiliary diseases: one plus one equals (sometimes) more than two. *Hepatology* 2004; 39: 604-7.
74. Stephens M, Smith NJ, Donnelly P. A new statistical method for haplotype reconstruction from population data. *Am J Hum Genet* 2001; 68: 978-89.
75. Drysdale CM, McGraw DW, Stack CB, Stephens JC, Judson RS, Nandabalan K, Arnold K, et al. Complex promoter and coding region beta 2-adrenergic receptor haplotypes alter receptor expression and predict *in vivo* responsiveness. *Proc Natl Acad Sci USA* 2000; 97: 10483-8.
76. The International HapMap Consortium. The International HapMap Project. *Nature* 2003; 426: 789-96.

Does the COX-1/COX-2 concept still hold?

Chris Hawkey

Institute of Clinical Research, Wolfson Digestive Diseases Centre, University Hospital, Nottingham, United Kingdom

Recognition that non-steroidal anti-inflammatory drugs were inhibitors of prostaglandin synthesis was critical to understanding of both their therapeutic activity and gastrointestinal pathology. In the stomach and duodenum, inhibition of prostaglandin synthesis abrogates defensive mechanisms such as mucosal blood flow, and mucus and bicarbonate secretion, and leads to the development of micro erosions that deepen ultimately to become ulcers as a consequence of acid peptic attack. Subsequently it has become clear that prostaglandin synthesis derives from two distinct but similar cyclooxygenase enzymes. The constitutive cyclooxygenase (COX)-1 is expressed in many tissues including the gastrointestinal tract. The inducible cyclooxygenase (COX)-2 becomes highly expressed under the influence of many factors such as cytokines and growth factors in tissue injury, inflammation and malignant transformation.

The COX-1/COX-2 hypothesis was that drugs which inhibit COX-2 would share the therapeutic active of NSAIDs but without their adverse effects.

Therapeutic activity

Numerous clinical trials have shown that COX-2 inhibitors relieve pain and inflammation in arthritis in a dose-dependent fashion with maximum effects that are usually not significantly different from NSAIDs. Thus, although some have suggested, contrary to the COX-1/COX-2 hypothesis, that COX-1 may contribute to symptoms in arthritis, this does not appear to be sufficiently great to have a measurable clinical impact.

Toxicity of COX-2 inhibitors and NSAIDs

Remarkably, acute studies show that even at very high doses (up to 10 times therapeutic) COX-2 inhibitors cause no demonstrable mucosal injury in healthy volunteers. Medium term endoscopy studies in patients show substantial reductions in ulceration compared to NSAIDs. In some, but not all, studies levels of ulceration have been similar to those observed on placebo. Because COX-2 is induced at the edge of ulcers, COX-2 inhibitors may in theory retard ulcer healing (like NSAIDs), and such an action could account for differences from placebo in longer term studies where the prevalence of ulcers could be hypothesized to rise because spontaneous ulcers heal less well. However, there are no direct data to suggest this is the case. In outcomes studies, the incidents of clinically significant ulcers or ulcer complications is reduced compared to NSAIDs. In most studies the reduction has been between 50% and 60% rather than the 75-85% that might be inferred from the 4 to 5 fold rise in ulcer complications caused by NSAIDs. Whether these values, and differences between drugs, arise by chance, because of study design or because COX-2 inhibitor outcome events have not fallen to truly placebo levels is not known but may become clearer from large ongoing studies in cancer where COX-2 inhibitors are compared to placebo.

Dyspepsia

The original COX-1/COX-2 hypothesis did not relate to dyspepsia. Nevertheless, high levels of dyspepsia on NSAIDs are sufficiently general that this may be a CLASS (and therefore mechanism) based effect. This argument is reinforced by data from COX-2 inhibitors which rather consistently seem to have level of dyspepsia that is greater than placebo but less than NSAIDs. Understanding the pharmacological mechanisms underlying this relationship may throw light on the pathogenesis of NSAID dyspepsia.

Thrombotic events

When patients present with NSAIDs associated ulcer bleeding, this may be because the NSAID causes ulcer formation or impairs haemostasis leading to bleeding. Equally, since vascular prostacyclin is recognised to be largely derived from the COX-2 enzyme, it is possible that COX-2 inhibitors could induce thrombosis. This issue came to a head in the VIGOR study where patients on naproxen had fewer thrombotic cardiovascular events than on rofecoxib. This could be attributed to a harmful effect of rofecoxib or of naproxen. Recent data suggest that the latter is dominant though the former may not be absent.

Cancer

Since COX-2 is induced in gastrointestinal cancers a development of the COX-1/COX-2 hypothesis predicts that Cox-2 inhibitors may prevent or reverse GI malignancy without harmful effects on normal mucosa. In animal and genetic models this has been shown in humans. However aspirin is also effective but is a COX-1 inhibitor. Understanding how aspirin prevents or reverses (pre) malignant processed in the gastrointestinal track will contribute to understanding of oncogenesis.

Practical prescribing

The COX-1/COX-2 hypothesis does not discount the influence of additional factors, and in fact acknowledges that NSAID ulcers have a prostaglandin dependent and an acid peptic dependent component. This would lead one to hypothesise that acid suppression and COX-2 inhibitor substitution might be complementary strategies in preventing ulcer disease. Recent data show that acid suppression very effectively diminishes ulcer development and dyspepsia in patients on COX-2 inhibitors at high risk of these two gastrointestinal problems.

IV

Abdominal problems in daily pratice

Free abdominal and/or retroperitoneal air. Clinical aspects

Guenter J. Krejs

Department of Internal Medicine, Medical University, Graz, Austria

The normal peritoneum is a well lubricated surface that allows a certain degree of movement of the intraabdominal organs. This is important for the hollow viscera, to allow normal motility with movement of intestinal contents from the esophagus to the anus. As in the pleural space, small amounts of fluids are secreted and resorbed; thus the normal peritoneal cavity contains very little fluid and so little gas that it is not detectable on normal imaging studies. Gas in the abdominal cavity is an important, and in most cases an alarming finding [1]. It is, in a large number of cases, the hallmark of an intraabdominal catastrophe, resulting from perforation of a hollow viscus. It is a characteristic of acute abdomen, and in the right clinical setting will need surgical intervention. However, there is also spontaneous and asymptomatic pneumoperitoneum with which the physician must be familiar in order to prevent unnecessary surgery. This chapter covers the clinical aspects of pneumoperitoneum; although the subsequent chapter covers the imaging aspects, there will be some images in this chapter to illustrate the clinical aspects.

Pneumoperitoneum in the context of acute abdomen

Acute abdomen is a condition of severe abdominal pain with laboratory signs of infection or inflammation, such as high white cell count and elevated C-reactive protein in serum; the physical exam shows a tender abdomen and typically a rebound phenomenon. In this clinical setting, free air in the abdomen will indicate perforation of a hollow viscus, as of a peptic ulcer in the stomach or duodenum, the gall bladder, large intestine or other part of the intestinal tract. Computer tomography often allows not only identification of free air in the peritoneum, but also of the origin, in the form of abnormal gastrointestinal wall structures (*e.g.* perforation with ischemic colitis or toxic megacolon). It is important to recognize extrusion of gas into the retroperitoneum *(figure 1)*.

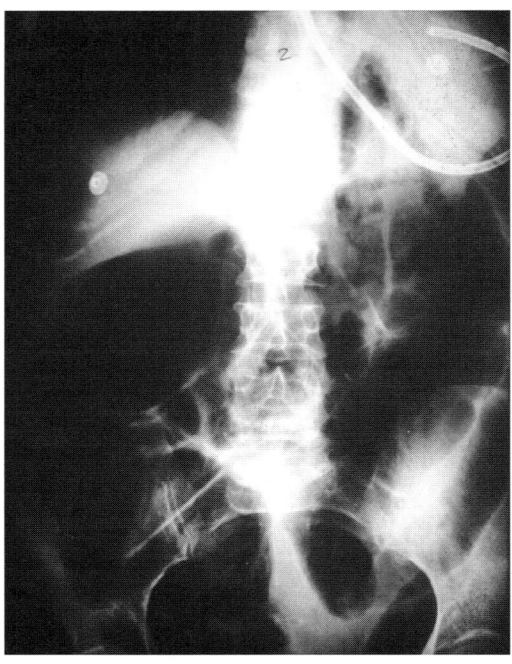

Figure 1. Flat plate of the abdomen in a 61-year-old female with several cardiovascular risk factors, admitted for acute myocardial infarction. In the ICU she developed abdominal pain and a distended abdomen. The large bowel is dilated down to the level of the descending colon. A nasogastric tube is in place. The gas collection up to the diaphragm to the left of the spine (nasogastric tube overlying in projection) cannot be attributed to a viscous or other normal structure in the GI tract. This was immediately recognized in the ICU by the consulting gastroenterologist. CT revealed retroperitoneal gas around the left kidney. Ischemic colitis with perforation in the distal descending colon was found upon laparotomy.

Pneumoperitoneum within the context of abnormal conditions of the wall of the gastrointestinal tract that are asymptomatic and usually do not require surgery

Asymptomatic or spontaneous pneumoperitoneum [2] can result from such conditions as small bowel diverticulosis and small intestinal or colonic pneumatosis. In pneumatosis, intramural cysts may rupture and lead to gas collection without symptoms and signs of peritonitis. *Figure 2* shows a routine chest X-ray on admission with an abundant amount of air under the diaphragm in a patient who was completely asymptomatic but had scleroderma. The flat plate of the abdomen *(figure 3)* gave the explanation, namely, intestinal pneumatosis with a string-of-pearls pattern of gas bubbles delineating the wall of a segment of the small bowel, this was confirmed with a barium study. Intestinal pneumatosis is a well-known complication in collagen vascular diseases. Colonic pneumatosis is often a disease of the elderly that may be associated with chronic pulmonary disease. Such patients may present with abdominal pain without peritoneal signs, or with hematochezia. Management allows for expectant observation and in some cases, high oxygen breathing. The latter will increase the gradient of gas partial pressures between the gas cysts and the surrounding tissue and so facilitate the disappearance of the gaseous cysts.

Post-procedure pneumoperitoneum

This can be a normal and expected finding, such as up to 1-2 days after laparotomy, or following laparoscopy or procedures to investige the patency of the female reproductive system with air insufflation into the fallopian tubes and hysterography. Physicians must, however, be cautious about attributing free air after laparotomy and laparoscopy to these

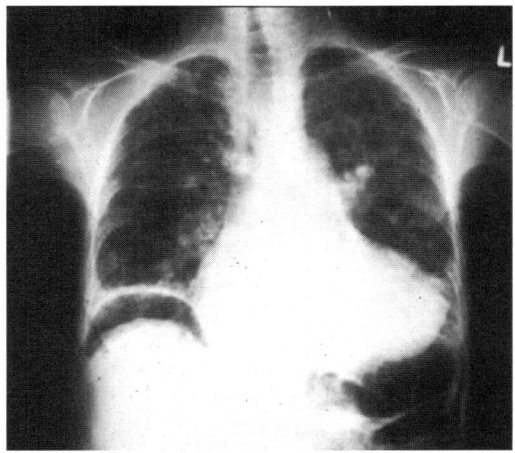

Figure 2. Free air under the right diaphragm in an asymptomatic patient with scleroderma.

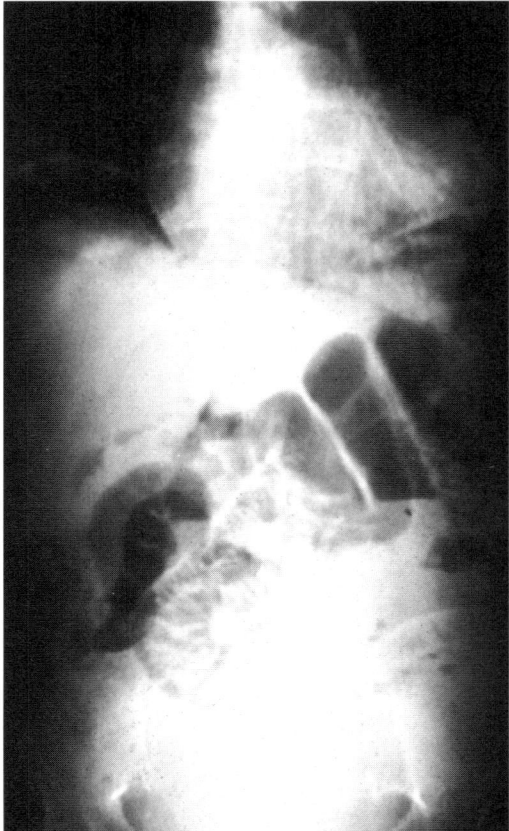

Figure 3. Same patient as in *figure 2*. The source of the free air is pneumatosis of the small bowel. Note the gas bubbles in a string-of-pearls pattern in the wall of the small bowel. Large-mouthed, gas-filled diverticula of the transverse colon, a typical finding in systemic sclerosis (true diverticula), are also seen.

procedures alone. In a recent case that resulted in litigation, severe abdominal pain and free air after gynecologcial laparoscopy and a procedure on one ovary was not due to gas insufflation during laparoscopy but to accidental injury to the colon. Because the symptoms had been ignored as "normal post-laparoscopy findings", emergency surgery with partial colectomy was required after two days. Peritoneal dialysis has also been recognized as sound for free abdominal air. The amounts of gas are usually small and pose no problems in the differential diagnosis.

Procedure-induced pneumoperitoneum as a result of iatrogenic perforation during gastroscopy, duodenoscopy, small-bowel suction biopsy, peritoneoscopy, colonoscopy, etc. needs to be recognized promptly *(figure 4)*. The risk of perforation during a diagnostic colonoscopy is deemed to be 1 in 10,000, during colonoscopy with polypectomy, 1 in 1,000 procedures. If the colonscopist recognizes the perforation, the patient may still be asymptomatic and immediate measures are necessary. In some cases, perforation can now be handled through the colonoscope using large clips or be repaired by laparoscopy instead of a standard laparotomy. One should certainly not wait until peritonitis develops. Hoping for a sealed-off perforation and self healing (with the help antibiotics) cannot be expected to be successful and would not be defensible as "standard management".

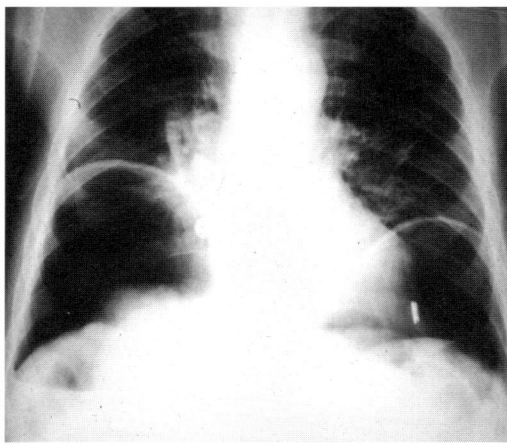

Figure 4. Large amounts of gas under both sides of the diaphragm following perforation during gastroscopy.

In some instances, iatrogenic pneumoperitoneum may allow observation without intervention. This happened to us in the beginning, when we used a neodymium YAG laser with an air jet. The air jet can dissect the wall of the stomach and enter the peritoneum without causing peritonitis. In such a case, the patient is to be managed expectantly, as with spontaneous pneumoperitoneum without peritonitis.

Special considerations

In a number of cases, sexual activity with vaginal insufflation (a form of cunnilingus) has been described as the cause of nonsurgical pneumoperitoneum [3]. The latter has also been described after scuba diving, when pneumoperitoneum may result from pulmonary interstitial emphysema and may present without pneumothorax or pneumomediastinum [4].

Pneumoperitoneum has also been reported in the context of status epilepticus, during which high gastrointestinal pressures develop because of high abdominal pressures with a closed glottis; this could induce lacerations of the mucosa and leakage of air into the peritoneum [5].

Pneumoperitoneum in association with mechanical ventilation has been recognized; it is generally but not always associated with pneumothorax and/or pneumomediastinum.

Tension pneumoperitoneum

This is a rare but life-threatening complication in critically ill patients [6]. A perforation of the digestive tract, be it after endoscopy or spontaneous due to localized necrosis of the bowel wall or ileus, may act like a valve. On inspiration, gas is sucked into the free peritoneal cavity. This leads to an increase in intraabdominal pressure (normally around 10 mmHg) up to 20-40 mmHg with resultant pulmonary and hemodynamic deterioration and cardiopulmonary arrest. The diagnosis should be made on clinical grounds (imaging studies show large amounts of free gas in the abdomen). Emergency decompression analogous to puncture and drainage of ascitic fluid is necessary.

References

1. Khan AN. Pneumoperitoneum. http://www.emedicine.com/radio/topic562htm
2. Zer M, Wolloch Y, Dinstman M. "Spontaneous" pneumoperitoneum. *Am J Proct Gast Col Rect Surg* 2004; 17: 35-8.
3. Mundhenke C, Mass N, Hilpert F, Jonat W. Sexual activity as cause for non-surgical pneumoperitoneum. *JSLS* 2001; 4: 297-300.
4. Rose DM, Jarczyk PA, Jarczyk PA. Spontaneous pneumoperitoneum after scuba diving. *JAMA*; 239, 223.
5. Richard C, Guiochon A, Rimalho A, Ricome JL, Auzepy P. Pneumoperitoneum complicating status epilepticus. *JAMA* 1981; 305 (27); 1651-2.
6. Ganter MT, Ganter CC, Schneemann M, Maggiorini M. Lebensbedrohliches Spannungs-Pneumoperitoneum. *Intensivmed* 2004; 42: 352-7.

New Developments in the Management of Benign GI Disorders.
D.J. Gouma, G.J. Krejs, G.N. Tytgat, Y. Finkel, eds. John Libbey Eurotext, Paris © 2004, pp. 99-108.

Treatment of intestinal obstruction: medical aspects

Jan Tack, M. Hiele, G. Coremans, L. Marchal, V. Moons

Department of Internal Medicine, Division of Gastroenterology, University Hospital Gasthuisberg, Catholic University of Leuven, Leuven, Belgium

Small bowel obstruction

Epidemiology

Intestinal obstruction is an important emergency for gastroenterologists and gastrointestinal surgeons. The most important causes of small bowel obstruction are postoperative adhesions (accounting for 50-75% of all cases), external herniae, benign and malignant neoplasms, and inflammatory bowel disease. Postoperative adhesions only exceptionally cause colonic obstruction. Colorectal cancer is responsible for 85-90% of all cases of colonic obstruction [1].

Pathophysioloy

When obstruction of the bowel occurs, stasis of intestinal fluid and of swallowed air occurs proximal to the site of obstruction. This leads to progressive distension of the bowel, increased pressure in the lumen, increased tension in the bowel wall, and hypovolemia. This is often accompanied by an inflammatory process in the bowel wall with edema, some of which leaks into the peritoneal cavity, producing ascites. As the intraluminal pressure increases, venous return is obstructed in the bowel wall, capillary filling is decreased, and arterial inflow begins to diminish with eventual ischemia. The mucosa, most sensitive to ischemia, is the first layer to become necrotic. This causes ulceration of the bowel wall, leading to bleeding and bacterial invasion of the bowel wall. Bacterial migration into the peritoneal cavity in the presence of ascites sets up the possibility of peritonitis developing. With continuing vascular compromise, full-thickness gangrene of the bowel develops, with subsequent perforation and peritonitis.

In the beginning of the previous century, it was shown that parenterally administered saline could prolong life in laboratory animals with intestinal obstruction. In the same period, reports of succesful application of intestinal suction in small bowel obstruction began to appear.

Conservative management

Regardless of the mode of therapy, early diagnosis remains the key to successful outcome of small bowel obstruction. Once diagnosed, fluid replacement and intestinal decompression should be started immediately. The presumed cause of small bowel obstruction is a major factor that will influence clinical management. Patients with obstruction due to an incarcerated inguinal hernia require surgical management. In those where there is no suspicion of strangulation and where the cause does not necessitate immediate surgery, conservative management can be attempted.

Several published series have established that surgery can be avoided in many patients with obstruction due to postoperative adhesions [2, 3]. Some authors distinguish partial from total obstruction. This is based on criteria like passage of flatus, presence of air in the colon on X-ray, passage of a small quantity of orally administered contrast, etc. The former is thought to have up to 80% chance of success with conservative management while the latter would only have a 10% to 15% success rate. However, in clinical practice, the distinction between both is often less clear and depends stronlgy on the timing of the assessment.

Miller *et al.* analysed the outcomes of 410 patients that were admitted with small bowel obstruction caused by adhesions. Thirty six percent was treated surgically. During follow-up, 34% of conservatively managed and 32% of surgically managed patients required a new hospitalisation. These figures show that conservative management is potentially successful, both in the short and in the long term [3].

Safety of conservative management

Of major concern in the management of small bowel obstruction is the status of the blood supply to the obstructed segment. With progressive of the distention obstructed bowel, compromise of the blood supply and full thickness gangrene may develop in a few hours. The risk of conservative management is not recognizing strangulation, which leads to increased morbidity and possibly mortality. Mortality rates for "simple" obstruction with intact blood supply are usually reported as less than 3%; with gangrene this rate rises to 10% or higher. Unfortunately, the clinical signs and symptoms of bowel necrosis are frequently absent or subtle or manifest themselves with some delay [4].

Very few data are available on the ouctome of conservative treatment management compared to immediate surgery. Mosley and Shoaib reported preliminary data of a randomised prospective study in which patients with small bowel obstruction due to adhesions were randomized to immediate surgery or conservative managements. The results have only been published in abstract form. The total group comprised 127 patients of which 63 were managed conservatively and 64 surgically. Of the conservatively managed group,

22 eventually required surgery and 2 died. Of the surgically treated group, four died. These data, in spite of their limitations, suggest that conservative management is not more risky than prompt surgery [5].

Long or short decompression tubes

Whether decompression is accomplished with simple naso-gastric suction or a long tube is not as important as is the need to begin suction at once. Once obstruction occurs, the pathophysiologic process may progress unless distension is reversed. A gastric decompression tube is easy to position and usually functions more easily than an intestinal decompression tube. A gastric tube does not use a mercury-filled bag at its tip, whereas small intestinal suction tubes usually have a mercury bag.

There are some theoretical advantages to suction beyond the pylorus, as this is closer to the site of obstruction which may allow a more eefficacious decompression. Moreover, the use of a small bowel decompression tube has the additional advantage that it can be used in a later phase contrast to administer contrast to perform enteroclysis.

A retropective analysis by Brolin *et al.* [6] evaluated the use of gastric or intestinal suction in 311 patients with 342 episodes of obstruction. They found no difference in outcome between both types of tube, but patients with a gastric suction tube were more likely to undergo surgery in the first 24 hours and the number of postoperative complications was higher in those treated with an intestinal tube.

In a retrospective analysis of small bowel obstruction managed conservatively in our unit, success was obtained in 63%. Of 56 patients treated with a nasogastric tube, 38% ultimately required surgery and 33% of these required segmental resection for strangulation. Of 14 patients treated with a nasointestinal tube, 21% ultimately required surgery and only 7% of these required segmental resection for strangulation [7].

Fleshner *et al.* performed a prospective randomised study on 55 patients with intestinal obstructions caused by adhesions. No significant differences were observed, but the group was really small and the positioning of the long tube beyond the pylorus did not always succeed [8].

Duration of conservative management

There is no consensus in the litterature on how long conservative management can be attempted. Recommendations vary between 12-24 hours and 5 days. Most authors propose 48 to 72 hours. A decision to end conservative management should be driven by the likelihood that an obstruction will resolve with ongoing management and by the risk of strangulation. In most cases where conservative management succeeds, this is within 48 and likelihood of success decreases beyond 72 hours, but is not zero. There are no certain clinical or biochemical indicators that allow to diagnose or exlude strangulation. Under certain circumstances (Crohn's disease with inflammatory obstruction, peritoneal metastases...) a longer conservative treatment period can be justified.

Conclusion

Both conservative management and surgery are important treatment options in the management of small bowel obstruction. Patients with irreversible causes or with suspected strangulation require surgery. According to the litterature, conservative management with intestinal decompression using nasogastric or nasointestinal tubes has a success rate of more than 50% in patients with potentially reversible causes and no signs of strangulation. The advantage of long endoscopically placed tubes is not established. Conservative management includes the risk of unrecognized strangulation for which no reliable diagnostic markers are available.

Acute colonic pseudo-obstruction

Definition and prevalence

The syndrome of acute colonic pseudo-obstruction was first described by Ogilvie in 1948. Ogilvie's syndrome is characterized by a massive dilation of the caecum and the right colon, in the absence of a distal mechanical obstruction. Since then, it has been recognized as a complication occurring in patients who underwent surgery and in patients with serious medical conditions. Ogilvie is associated with an underlying disease in 95 percent of patients. Most often, the dilatation of the right colon is associated with a simultaneous pseudo-obstruction of the small intestine, which is less severe.

Ogilvie's syndrome is a relatively rare condition, but since the original description more than 500 cases were described in literature. It has been estimated that this complication occurs in approximately 0.1% of the patients undergoing surgery, in approximately 0.05% of the patients admitted for trauma and in 0.3% of critically ill patients with burns [9, 10]. Elderly patients have a higher risk of developing acute colonic pseudo-obstruction [11].

Clinical features

Ogilvie is more common in men and in patients over the age of 60. The symptoms associated with colonic pseudo-obstruction occur as a consequence of a progressive dilatation of the right colon. Initially a painless abdominal distention may occur, followed by nausea and vomiting. Abdominal pain is generally mild and constant. Cessation of bowel movements is often present, but almost half of the patients continue to pass flatus. Occasionally, diarrhea may accompany the syndrome.

The most obvious clinical finding is abdominal distention. In case of massive dilatation of the colon, mild rebound tenderness can be present. Bowel sounds may be normal, hyperactive or clangorous. In most of the cases, the abdomen is tympanic, although bowel sounds are present in almost 90 percent of patients.

Peritoneal signs are absent in the early stages of the disease. If present, they suggest impending perforation. A low-grade fever may also be present. There are no pathognomonic physical or laboratory findings.

Complications

The most severe complication of colonic pseudo-obstruction, with a high mortality rate, is a colonic perforation and ischemic necrosis caused by progressive massive dilatation. When a perforation occurs, this is usually at the level of the caecum. A diameter of the caecum on abdominal X-rays of 12 cm or more indicates imminent perforation. Perforation should be suspected in case of a clinically quiet abdomen, increasing fever and progressive elevation of the leukocyte count.

Diagnosis and differential diagnosis

Laboratory tests may show increased blood leukocytes, and disturbances in electrolyte levels such as hypokalemia, hyponatremia, hypocalcemia or hypomagnesemia.

If leucocytosis is present, it is not due to uncomplicated obstruction, but to an underlying disease or to a perforation.

Acute colonic pseudo-obstruction has to be differentiated from mechanical colonic obstruction caused by sigmoidvolvulus, tumors, benign strictures or fecal impaction. Additional differential diagnosis include toxic megacolon, ischemic colitis, typhlitis and chronic idiopathic intestinal pseudo-obstruction.

A plain abdominal X-ray will demonstrate dilatation of the right colon (caecum > 9 cm), most often with an abrupt end at the hepatic or splenic flexure. Haustral markings are normal.

A prone lateral X-ray of the rectum demonstrating gaseous distention of the rectum may add to the diagnosis. Gaseous distention of the rectum does not occur in patients with structural obstructive lesions and is suggestive for pseudo-obstruction [12]. Although the colon is usually devoid of air-fluid levels, they may be present in dilated loops of small intestine.

An enema with water-soluble contrast medium may further aid in diagnosing colonic pseudo-obstruction and in excluding mechanical obstruction and toxic megacolon.

Its sensitivity and specificity is higher than that of plain abdominal X-ray and history. Colonoscopy has both diagnostic and therapeutic possibilities and is considered a safe procedure in the setting of acute colonic pseudo-obstruction.

Pathogenesis

The pathogenesis and pathophysiology of Ogilvie's syndrome remain unknown. Some indications suggest an imbalance of the inhibitory sympathetic and the excitatory parasympathetic innervation of the distal colon, leading to a functional obstruction. Excessive large bowel parasympathetic suppression, rather than sympathetic hyperactivity, has been put forward as the underlying mechanism [13]. A variety of abdominal and extra-abdominal conditions associated with acute colonic pseudo-obstruction has been reported *(table I)* [9, 14].

Table I. Conditions associated with acute colonic pseudo-obstruction

- Trauma (non-surgical)
- Surgery (abdominal, gynecologic, orthopedic, urologic)
- Inflammatory processes (pancreatitis, cholecystitis, appendicitis...)
- Toxic megacolon (IBD, pseudomembranous colitis...)
- Malignancy
- Radiation therapy
- Drugs (narcotis, antidepressants, phenothiazines, clonidine, anticholinergics, corticosteroids, theophylline)
- Cardiovascular disease
- Neurologic disease
- Respiratory failure
- Metabolic disease (electrolyte and acid-base imbalance, diabetes, hypothyroidism, alcoholism, uremia, lead poisoning)
- Burns
- Retroperitoneal hemorrhage
- Mesenteric ischemia

Treatment

The goals of therapy are to avoid perforation and to temporise until the syndrome runs its course.

Treatment consists of conservative measures, removal of precipitants, colonoscopic decompression, surgical caecostomy and laparotomy. Although numerous cases have been reported in the literature, controlled clinical trials are lacking.

• A trial of **conservative measures** alone is appropriate in patients who lack significant abdominal pain, who have no signs of peritonitis and who have underlying factors that are potentially reversible. Conservative measures include correction of fluid and electrolyte imbalance, cessation of sedative, narcotic and anticholinergic drugs, treatment of underlying systemic medical conditions, optimization of tissue oxygenation and withholding oral intake [9]. Maximization of physical activity and positional changes can be useful [15]. Conservative measures also include intestinal decompression using nasogastric suction and insertion of a rectal canula through a rigid rectoscope. Gentle enemas can be used, but with much care not to cause perforation. Oral laxatives are generally not helpful, and lactulose should be avoided as it may promote intraluminal accumulation of gas. The patient should be mobilized or periodically turned from side to side and also placed prone.

• A second step is the use of **pharmacologic agents** which might stimulate the colonic motility.

A few medications have been used in recent studies.

1. *Erythromycin.* This medication stimulates smooth muscle contraction by binding to motilin receptors in the intestine. It has strong prokinetic properties in the upper gut. Anecdotal reports exist of three patients treated succesfully with erythromycin either orally (250 mg QID for 10 days) of intravenously (250 mg in 250 ml of normal saline every eight hours for three days).

2. *Cisapride.* It acts by enhancing the release of acetylcholine in the myenteric plexus of the gut wall and induces colonic contraction and shortens colonic transit time. There is only one report of one single patient who has been treated succesfully with cisapride (10 mg IV every four hours for four doses, followed by 10 mg PO TID). Cisapride may be complicated by cardiac arythmias.

3. *Neostigmine.* This is an acethylcholinesterase inhibitor acting by competing with acetylcholine for attachement to acetylcholinesterase at sites of cholinergic transmission. A recent study [16] did show a complete clinical resolution of large bowel distention in 26 of 28 patients (93%). Time to flatus varied from 30 seconds to 10 minutes after administration of 2.5 mg IV over 3 minutes. No complications of adverse effects were noted.

Other studies performed by Ponec [17], Stephenson *et al.* [18] (2.5 mg IV neostigmine as a slow injection over 3 minutes alone) and Turegano-Fuentes *et al.* [19] (2.5 mg in 100 ml of normal saline over 60 minutes) did show a rapid and satisfactory clinical and radiological decompression of the large bowel in a high percent of patients. In most patients the response was durable. The most frequent adverse effect that was seen was mild to moderate crampy abdominal pain, which was transient. The most important possible complication is symptomatic bradycardia requiring atropine, although the appearance is very low. Other side-effects noted were excessive salivation and vomiting.

In addition to those medications anecdotal success has been reported with ganglionic blockers (guanethidine), ganglionic stimulants (nicotine patch) and epidural anesthesia (to provide sympathetic blockade). Naloxone may be useful in opioid-induced acute colonic pseudo-obstruction. Conservative treatment without colonoscopy may result in a resolution of the dilatation in 53 to 96% within 3 to 6 days [9, 20].

• **Endoscopic decompression of the colon** is indicated when the colonic diameter exceeds 12 cm, when dilatation persists for more than 48 to 72 hours under supportive measures, and in the presence of progressive dilatation or clinical deterioration. But there is no exact colonic diameter that mandates decompression.

Uncontrolled studies suggest that colonoscopic decompression is a safe procedure [21]. Standard colon cleansing before colonoscopy is omitted by patients with Ogilvie's syndrome. Stool in the distal colon can be removed by small-volume saline enemas. Successful colonoscopic decompression is achieved in 60% to 90% of the patients with Ogilvie's syndrome, but recurrence may occur in 20% to 45%. Insertion of a multi-fenestrated decompression tube during colonoscopy may help to avoid rapid recurrence. It is, however, a laborious procedure with a potentially higher risk when the tube is dragged along by the colonoscope. Moreover, the tube can become occluded with solid fecal material. However, the reported perforation rate is less than 2% with morbidity and mortality rates of only 3 and 1% respectively [16-19, 22-26].

Colonoscopic decompression only causes a small decrease in cecal size [26]. The clinical benefit of colonoscopic decompression has been demonstrated in patients with acute pseudo-obstruction. But the early clinical improvement does not necessarily correlate with radiografic changes in caecal diameter [26].

Decompression may also consist of percutaneous tube cecostomy. This procedure is more invasive, involving endoscopic and radiographic approach and is usually reserved for those who fail initial endoscopic decompression. This procedure has a mortality rate of 15%.

- **Surgery** is reserved to patients in which medical management and endoscopic decompression were unsuccessful or by clinical signs indicating impending or actual cecal perforation.

The type of surgery is depending upon the finding during the surgery.

1. ***Surgical caecostomy*** is indicated when endoscopic decompression was unsuccessful. In the absence of ischemia or perforation, a simple surgical caecostomy can be performed under local anesthesia. As an alternative, a percutaneous caecostomy can be accomplished by a Seldinger puncture guided by laparoscopy, ultrasonography or radiography [27]. Catheter caecostomy requires vigorous postoperative tube to ensure adequate function and minimal morbidity. Abdominal wall cellulitis and sepsis have been reported as complications.

2. Patients who have a perforated bowel, need a ***total colectomy, ileostomy or a Hartmann procedure***. Decompressive transverse colostomies and diverting ileostomies produce a mortality rate up to 40% in absence of colonic necrosis, rising to 50% in presence of colonic necrosis and peritonitis. Exploratory laparotomy is indicated in patients with massive caecal distention presenting with pneumoperitoneum development of peritonitis, respiratory failure and diagnostic uncertainty.

Reported overall mortality rate of surgical procedures in patients with acute colonic pseudo-obstruction is 10-15%.

Prognosis

In spite of optimal management, mortality rates of 3% to 50% have been reported. Risk factors are old age, underlying diseases, caecal size and delay of adequate therapy. Early diagnosis and clinical awareness in case of painless abdominal distention in a patient with a predisposing condition are important in avoiding significant morbidity and mortality.

References

1. Aufses AH. Treatment of intestinal obstruction: suction *versus* surgery. In: *Emergencies in gastroetnerology and hepatology*. Leuven University Press, 1996: 115-8.
2. Wolfson PJ, Bauer JJ, Gelernt IM, Kreel I, Aufses AH Jr. Use of the long tube in the management of patients with small-intestinal obstruction due to adhesions. *Arch Surg* 1985; 120: 1001-6.
3. Miller G, Boman J, Shrier I, Gordon PH. Natural history of patients with adhesive small bowel obstruction. *Br J Surg* 2000; 87: 1240-7.
4. Sarr MG, Bulkley GB, Zuidema GD. Preoperative recognition of intestinal strangulation obstruction: prospective evaluation of diagnostic capability. *Am J Surg* 1983; 145: 176-82.
5. Mosley GJ, Shoaib A. Operative *versus* conservative management of adhesional intestinal obstruction. *Br J Surg* 2000; 87: 368 (abstract).
6. Brolin RE, Krasna MJ, Mast BA. Use of tubes and radiographs in the management of small bowel obstruction. *Ann Surg* 1987; 206: 126-33.
7. Hiele M, Coremans G, Marchal L. Intestinale obstructie: conservatieve aanpak. *Tijdschrift voor geneeskunde* 2003; 59: 461-5.
8. Fleshner PR, Siegman MG, Slater GI, *et al*. A prospective, randomized trial of short *versus* long tubes in adhesive small-bowel obstruction. *Am J Surg* 1995; 170: 366-70.
9. Vanek WV, Al-Salti M. Acute pseudo-obstruction of the colon (Ogilvie's syndrome): an anlysis of 400 cases. *Dis Colon Rectum* 1986; 29: 203-10.
10. Kadesky K, Purdue GF, Hunt JL. Acute pseudo-obstruction in critically ill patients with burns. *J Burn Care Rehabil* 1995; 16: 132-5.
11. Jetmore AB, Timmcke AE, Gathbright JB, Hicks TC, Ray JE, Baker JW. Ogilvie's syndrome: colonosocpic decompresion and analysis of predisposing factors. *Dis Colon Rectum* 1992; 35: 1135-42.
12. Low VH. Colonic pseudo-osbtructin: value of prone lateraal view of the rectum. *Abdom Imaging* 1995; 20: 531-3.
13. Hutchinson R, Griffiths C. Acute colonic pseudo-obstruction: a pharmacological approach. *Ann R Coll Surg Engl* 1992; 74: 364-7.
14. Feldman RA, Karl RC. Diagnosis and treeatment of Ogilvie's syndrome after lumbar spinal surgery. Report of three cases. *J Neurosurg* 1992; 76: 1012-6.
15. Michael J. H. Management of Ogilvie's syndrome. *Gastrointest Endosc* 1997; 45: 540.
16. Gino T, Trevisani, Hyman NH. Neostigmine. Safe and effective treatment for acute colonic pseudo-obstruction. *Dis Colon Rectum* 2000; 43: 599-603.
17. Ponec RJ, Saunders, *et al*. Neostigmine for the treatment of acute colonic pseudo-obstruction. *N Engl J Med* 1999; 341: 137.
18. Stephenson BM, Morgan AR, *et al*. Ogilvie's syndrome: a new approach to an old problem. *Dis Colon Rectum* 1995; 40: 1353-7.
19. Turegano-Fuentez *et al*. 1997.
20. Sloyer AF, Panella VW, Demas BE, *et al*. Ogilvie's syndrome: successful management without colonoscopy. *Dig Dis Sci* 1988; 33: 1391-6.
21. Fiorito JJ, Schoen RE, Brandt LJ. Pseudo-obstruction associated with colonic ischemia: successful managementt with colonoscopic decompression. *Am J Gastroenterol* 1991; 86: 1472-6.
22. Nano D, Prindiville T, Pauby M, Chow H, Ross K, Trudeau W. Colonsoscopic therapy of actue pseudo-obstruction of the colon. *Am J Gastroenterol* 1987; 82: 145-8.
23. Sariego J, Matsumoto T, Kerstein MD. Colonoscopically guided tube decompression in Ogilvie's syndrome. *Dis Colon Rectum* 1991; 34: 720-2.
24. Stephenson KR, Rodriguez-Bigas MA. Decompression of the large intestine in Ogilvie's syndrome by a colonoscopically placed long intestinal tube. *Surg Endosc* 1994; 8: 116-7.
25. Strodel WE, Brothers TC. Colonoscopic decompression of pseudo-obstruction and volvulus. *Surg Clin North Am* 1989; 69: 1327-35.

26. Pham TN, Bard CC, Chu P. Radiographic changes after colonoscopic decompression for acute pseudo-obstruction. *Dis Colon Rectum* 1999; 42: 1586-91.
27. Van Sonnenberg E, Varney RR, Casoa G, *et al.*. Percutaneous cecostomy for Ogilvie syndrome: laboratory observations and clinical experience. *Radiology* 1990; 175: 679-82.

V

Gastrointestinal infections

Should *Helicobacter pylori* therapy be performed in all infected individuals?

Peter Malfertheiner

Otto-von-Guericke-University Magdeburg, Department of Gastroenterology, Hepatology and Infectious Diseases, Magdeburg, Germany

Intensive research for more than twenty years has well defined the clinical relevance of *H. pylori* infection and clarified many of the underlying basic mechanisms responsible for various clinical manifestations and outcomes. To translate the scientific progress into clinical practice updated recommendations of whom and how to treat were released [1] *(tables I and II)*. These recommendations are still quite complex and supported by different levels of scientific strength according to the nature of the *H. pylori* associated diseases as well as the quality of studies targeting the relative issues. The limitation is that current indications for *H. pylori* therapy in clinical practice are directed to cure the complications of the infection rather than to prevent any of them.

Successful treatment of patients by *H. pylori* eradication with overt disease such as peptic ulcer disease with or without further complications or MALT lymphoma in early stage has convinced even the most sceptical and these indications are no longer a matter of debate. There has in addition been an important move forward by considering other areas for *H. pylori* therapy. Among these eradication therapy has been found appropriate also in patients with functional dyspepsia. Even primary prevention is considered in situations such as prior to NSAID exposure. Many reports also indicate that *H. pylori* eradication has additional benefits in systemic extragastric diseases. In particular cure of some skin diseases, joint diseases and immuno thrombocytopenia by *H. pylori* eradication has been reported by several authors. However adequate randomized controlled studies for definitive proof are lacking in these conditions [2].

The critical question, however, is why should we astain from therapy in some circumstances and why not cure everyone in whom *H. pylori*-infection is detected. The question to follow is how proactive should we search for *H. pylori* infection. The current two main hurdles against a general screen and treat strategy are i) the still rather complex standard

Table I. A. Strongly recommended indications for *H. pylori* eradication according to Maastricht 2-2000 (from [1])

Indication	Scientific evidence
DU/GU (active or not, including complicated PUD)	1
MALToma	2
Atrophic gastritis	2
Post gastritis cancer resection	3
Patients who are first degree relatives of gastric cancer patients	3
Patients wishes (after full consultation with their physician)	4

Table I. B. Advisable indications and relevant statements according to Maastricht 2-2000 (from [1])

Indication	Scientific evidence
Functional dyspepsia	
• *H. pylori* eradication is an appropriate option	2
• This leads to long-term symptom improvement in a subset of patients	2
GERD *H. pylori* **eradication:**	
• Is not associated with GERD development in most cases	3
• Does not exacerbate existing GERD	3
H. pylori should be eradicated, though, in patients requiring long-term profound acid suppression	3
NSAIDs *H. pylori* **eradication:**	
• Reduces the incidence of ulcer, given prior to NSAID use	2
• Alone, is insufficient to prevent recurrent ulcer bleeding in high risk	2
NSAID users	
• Does not enhance healing of GU or DU in patients receiving antisecretory therapy who continue to take NSAIDs	1
H. pylori and NSAIDs/aspirin are independent risk factors for PUD	2

Table II. Arguments for *H. pylori* therapy in all infected

- *H. pylori* induces chronic gastritis in all infected subjects.
- *H. pylori* is the critical factor in peptic ulcer disease and gastric cancer.
- Predisposing factors are helpful to identify persons at increased risk – however not yet in practical use !

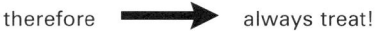

- *H. pylori* eradication heals ulcer disease and has the potential to prevent any kind of *H. pylori* related complication.
- Side effects can be controlled.
- Risks outweighed by benefit.
- Serious long-term conditions not expected.

therapy with considerable chance of failure, side effects and induction of antibiotic resistance; ii) the fear to induce harmful long term consequences, such as GERD and related complications.

The benefit of a global screen and treat strategy for *H. pylori* eradication is that in contrast to selected indications this approach bears the chance to prevent all or most of the potential harmful consequences induced by *H. pylori* with the most important aim being gastric cancer prevention.

H. pylori and gastric cancer: background and rationale for prevention

Gastric cancer is the second most frequent cause of cancer-related deaths on a global scale. Outside Japan diagnostic strategies have not been successful to increase the detection of early gastric cancer which is a curable condition. We continue to be faced with the clinical burden of more than 80% of patients with gastric cancer detected in an advanced stage and with dismal prognosis. The discovery of *H. pylori* and the identification of its association with gastric cancer provide us with the unique opportunity of a new management approach to get control over this disease.

Where is the evidence?

Extensive seroepidemiological and biological studies (in humans and animal models) have identified *H. pylori* as the most critical risk factor for the development of gastric cancer. Two recent carefully performed epidemiological studies that avoided some of the previous methodological pitfalls established the risk at much higher levels than previously thought of [3, 4]. In one of these two studies the concluding statement was that *H. pylori* is to be considered a *"conditio sine qua non"* for gastric cancer development.

Several models favouring either sequential or more direct histomorphological changes preceding gastric cancer have been proposed. The molecular mechanisms underlying various steps from *H. pylori* induced chronic inflammation of the gastric mucosa to fullblown neoplasia are increasingly elucidated (for review [5]). The activation of defined epithelial cell receptors (*i.e.* c-met receptor) by *H. pylori* as recently shown has added to our understanding of how *H. pylori* induces cell proliferation and other cellular mechanisms involved in carcinogenesis [6]. Virulence factors of *H. pylori* (CagA, VacA) on one side and genetically determined host response, IL 1-β polymorphisms and other polymorphisms of proinflammatory cytokines are key elements tracing the route in gastric carcinogenesis [7, 8]. Most importantly there are also two clinical trials published recently that lend further support to the role of *H. pylori* therapy in gastric cancer prevention [9, 10].

The critical issue is the point of no return

The critical question is whether *H. pylori* eradication is still effective in arresting the progress or even reverse the pathway embarked towards carcinogenesis in the presence of established preneoplastic changes. Atrophy and intestinal metaplasia (IM) in particular if corpus dominant are considered as preneoplasia and carry an increased gastric cancer risk. Atrophy and intestinal metaplasia are accompanied by several molecular alterations known for their contribution in gastric carcinogenesis (*i.e.* increased telomerase activity, microsatellite instability, accumulation and mutation of *p53*, overexpression of Cox2 and cyclin D2, plus several others).

The effect of *H. pylori* eradication on the reversibility of atrophy is highly controversial as reported in a recent review by Hojo [11]. Concerning atrophy, 11 of 25 authors reported some improvement, 13 authors found no significant change and one reported even a worsening of the atrophic changes. Data on IM is more consistent with only four of 28 studies describing any improvement. There are several shortcomings in the available studies either due to biopsy sampling bias, inconsistency in grading atrophy among studies and differences in the selection of the study population. At the present state, one is tempted to speculate that reversibility of preneoplastic lesions is unlikely to occur, but rather progression in some patients is observed in spite of successful eradication as recently indicated [10].

In the study of Wong *et al.* only those with chronic gastritis and preneoplastic changes progressed to cancer, whereas those with chronic active gastritis did not [10].

From studies on reversibility of preneoplastic lesions we can conclude i) start treating as early as possible!, ii) continue to follow patients with preneoplastic changes in spite of the infection being cured.

What is the clinical consequence at present?

We have recognized *H. pylori* as an essential factor in the pathogenesis of gastric cancer, we have non invasive tools available for easy detection and a seven day-therapy for cure of the *H. pylori* infection. We therefore have the premises to intervene early in the cascade of events towards gastric cancer using a screen and treat policy *(table II)*.

However the health economic burden for a screen and treat policy appears unproportionally high, taking into consideration that more than three billions of people on a worldwide scale would need to undergo a therapy with 80% eradication success rate. If the hypothesis is correct that gastric cancer prevention through *H. pylori* eradication could be achieved by around 70%, this is counterbalanced by billions of people who would never develop gastric cancer inspite being infected *H. pylori*. The figures however would change if all other potential *H. pylori* related complications can be prevented.

Another critical issue is certainly the current therapy based on two antibiotics plus PPI, which has still a high cost and is faced with problems such as antibiotic resistance induction. Therefore, at this stage, the preventive strategy should target selected populations and patients groups at higher risk as outlined in our recent European Consensus Conference [1]. However, we should not stop here in our engagement to fight gastric cancer by adopting *H. pylori* eradication, but elaborate on further strategies which will need to include cheaper and easier to handle therapies.

What are the concerns?

Risk of antibiotic resistance induction

Any use of antimicrobials constitutes a risk for antimicrobial resistance. For *H. pylori* the resistance mechanism is predominantly mutation. The macrolide spread of resistant bacteria is currently more restricted to Western societies, whereas metronidazole resistance is high around the world. Amoxicillin resistance is still exceptional.

For extended use of triple therapies as current standard it is therefore crucial to know the geographical-regional resistance pattern.

Risk of the development of gastro-oesophageal diseases

Reviews of case control studies suggest that *H. pylori*-infection is less common in patients with GERD compared to controls [12]. Evidence supporting the proposition that *H. pylori* eradication leads to GERD symptoms and/or erosive esophagitis is conflicting, however. Post hoc analysis of large trials on patients cured for peptic ulcer disease revealed no indication that *H. pylori* eradication for ulcer disease lead to development of erosive esophagitis or new symptomatic GERD [13, 14]. There is also no worsening of symptoms in patients with pre-existing GERD. The results were similar for studies conducted in patients with pre-existing GERD [15-17] or in the general population [18]. Overall, therefore, there is little randomised controlled trial evidence to suggest that *H. pylori* eradication leads to GERD symptoms.

There appears to be an inverse association also between *H. pylori*-infection (cagA type) and GERD or Barrett's esophagus. Case control studies have also suggested that CagA carrying *H. pylori* strains are less prevalent in patients with esophageal adenocarcinoma [19, 20], although this has not been a universal observation [22]. The uncertainty in the data with a slightly preponderings evidence of an inverse association between *H. pylori* and esophageal adenocarcinoma do not allow to draw any causal implications and in any case the risk of gastric adenocarcinoma outweighs by far any theoretical benefit in terms of protection from esophageal adenocarcinoma.

Current strategies in *H. pylori* management

Endoscopy based strategies: should be employed whenever a firm diagnosis is mandatory.

Test and treat

The most accepted non-invasive management strategy is a so called *Test and Treat Strategy*. This is a symptom-related strategy applicable in restricted conditions. In this strategy non-invasive *H. pylori* testing (C13 Urea breath test, stool antigen assay) is undertaken as the first line investigation in young people (< 45 years) who present with dyspepsia without alarm symptoms and no familial history of malignancy. Those who are *H. pylori* positive subsequently receive an eradication therapy while those who are not infected receive empirical symptomatic treatment with PPI. Such a strategy has advantages in reducing the endoscopy workload and is cost-effective in populations with a background prevalence of infection > 20%.

Search and treat

Serves two purposes: i) searching for patients with chronic antisecretory therapy (PPI, H2RA) for dyspeptic symptoms who may be naive *H. pylori* positive ulcer patients: eradication will resolve the problem in these patients; ii) search for *H. pylori* infection in first degree relatives of patients with gastric cancer and other patient groups at increased risk. This strategy may also be extended to populations at increased gastric cancer risk. The diagnostic method may be non invasive or endoscopy-based depending on the clinical setting and scenarios.

Screen and treat

Would confer the optimal chance to all people in the world but has still limitations because of the current therapy and financial restrictions.

How to treat

The currently recommended therapy for eradication is a short, seven day-combination of a PPI (standard dose bid) with clarithromycin and either amoxicillin or metronidazole, known as triple therapy. Intention to treat analyses have confirmed that triple therapy achieves successful eradication in ~ 80%. The choice between combining clarithromycin (C) with either amoxicillin (CA) or metronidazole (CM) is difficult. Gastrointestinal side effects, particularly diarrhoea are more frequent when a CA combination is used (20% *versus* 10%). CA is the treatment of choice in regions with high levels of primary metronidazole resistance [1]. An overview on how to proceed with *H. pylori* eradication therapies in *table III*.

Table III. Standard 7-day-therapy for *H. pylori* infection

	PPI standard bid	Clarithromycin	Metronidazole	Amoxicillin
Option 1		2 × 500 mg		2 × 1000 mg
Option 2		2 × 500 (250) mg	2 × 400 mg or 2 × 500 mg	

Above always in combination with a twice daily Standard-Dose of PPI (alternatives: omeprazole 2 × 20 mg, lansoprazole 2 × 30 mg, pantoprazole 2 × 40 mg, rabeprazole 2 × 20 mg, esomeprazole 2 × 20 mg)

Second-line-therapy for *H. pylori* infection (7 days)

Bismuth	PPI standard dose Bd.	Tetracycline	Metronidazole
Bismutsubcitrate 4 × 100 mg or Bismut-subsalicylate 4 × 600 mg	Omeprazole 2 × 20 mg, Lansoprazole 2 × 30 mg, Pantoprazole 2 × 40 mg, Rabeprazole 2 × 20 mg, Esomeprazole 2 × 20 mg	4 × 500 mg	3 × 500 mg

Options in case of repeated failures

- PPI-amoxicillin high dose 10 to 14 days.
- PPI-amoxicillin-rifabutin- (or levofloxacin) 7 to 10 days.
- PPI-bismuth-tetracycline-furazolidone 7 days.
- **Resistance testing in specialized laboratories is the best option and recommended whenever possible.**

Treatment failure is frequently a result of either poor patient compliance (improved with the advent of shorter treatment duration) or antibiotic or PPI resistance [22]. The issue of antimicrobial primary resistance has become increasingly important. It has been estimated that the worldwide prevalence of primary resistance to metronidazole and clarithromycin is in the order of 20-70% and 1-12% respectively. These figures vary dramatically by region. Amoxicillin resistance appears extremely uncommon. Secondary resistance to metronidazole has been demonstrated in 60-70% and to clarithromycin in 30-50%. Despite this, second line treatments have been developed which offer eradication rates of 70-80% and which may be employed without necessitating culture and antibiotic sensitivity testing. If second line therapy fails, it is advisable to repeat a gastroscopy and to obtain mucosal samples for culture and sensitivity analysis as otherwise re-treatment is unlikely to be successful [22, 23]. The development of new practical and easy to handle drugs to control the world wide infection even in the asymptomatic populations with the aim of disease prevention remains an ongoing challenge.

References

1. Malfertheiner P, Megraud F, O'Morain C, Hungin APS, Jones R, Axon A, Graham DY, Tytgat GNJ. Current concepts in the management of *Helicobacter pylori* infection – The Maastricht 2-2000 Consensus Report. *Aliment Pharmacol Ther* 2002; 16: 167-80.
2. Howden CW. A test-and-treat strategy is obsolete in primary care. In: Hunt RH, Tytgat GNJ, eds. H. pylori – *basic mechanisms to clinical cure*. Kluwer Academic Publishers, 2002: 297-300.
3. Ekström M, et al. *H. pylori* in gastric cancer established by CagA immunoblot as a marker of past infection. *Gastroenterology* 2001; 121: 784-91.
4. Brenner H, Arndt V, Stegmaier C, Ziegler H, Rothenbacher D. Is *H. pylori* infection a necessary condition for noncardia gastric cancer? *Am J Epidemiol* 2004; 159: 252-8.
5. Nardone G, Rocco A, Malfertheiner P. *Helicobacter pylori* and molecular events in precancerous gastric lesions. *Aliment Pharmacol Ther* 2004; 20: 261-70.
6. Churin Y, Al-Ghoul L, Kepp O, Meyer TF, Birchmeier W, Naumann M. *Helicobacter pylori* CagA protein targets the c-Met receptor and enhances the motogenic response. *J Cell Biol* 2003; 28: 249-55.
7. El Omar EM, Rabkin CS, Gammon MD, Vaughan TL, Risch HA, Schoenberg JB, Stanford JL, Mayne ST, Goedert J, Blot WJ, Fraumeni JF Jr, Chow WH. Increased risk of noncardia gastric cancer associated with proinflammatory cytokine gene polymorphisms. *Gastroenterology* 2003; 124: 1193-201.
8. Figueiredo C, Machado JC, Pharoah P, *et al. Helicobacter pylori* and interleukin 1 genotyping: an opportunity to identify high-risk individuals for gastric carcinoma. *J Natl Cancer Instit* 2002; 94: 1680-7.
9. Uemura N, Okamoto S, Yamamoto S, *et al. H. pylori* infection and the development of gastric cancer. *N Engl J Med* 2001; 345: 784-9.
10. Wong BCY, Lam SK, Wong WM, Chen JS, Zhen TT, *et al. H. pylori* eradication to prevent gastric cancer in a high-risk region of China. *JAMA* 2004; 291: 187-94.
11. Hojo M, Miwa H, Ohkusa T, Ohkura R, Kurosawa A, Sato N. Alteration of histological gastritis after cure of *Helicobacter pylori* infection. *Aliment Pharmacol Ther* 2002; 16: 1923-32.
12. Raghunath A, Hungin AP, Wooff D, Childs S. Prevalence of *Helicobacter pylori* in patients with gastro-oesophageal reflux disease: systematic review. *Br Med J* 2003; 326: 737.
13. Laine L, Sugg J. Effect of *H. pylori* eradication on development of erosive esophagitis and gastroesophageal reflux disease symptoms: a post hoc analysis of eight double-blind prospective studies. *Am J Gastroenterol* 2002; 97: 2992-7.
14. Malfertheiner P. *H. pylori* eradication does not exacerbate gastro-oesophageal reflux disease. *Gut* 2004; 53: 312-3.
15. Moayyedi P, Bardhan C, Young L, Dixon MF, Brown L, Axon AT. *Helicobacter pylori* eradication does not exacerbate reflux symptoms in gastroesophageal reflux disease. *Gastroenterology* 2001; 121: 1120-6.
16. Schwizer W, Thumshirn M, Dent J, Guldenschuh I, Menne D, Cathomas G, Fried MW, *et al. Helicobacter pylori* and symptomatic relapse of gastro-oesophageal reflux disease: a randomised controlled trial. *Lancet* 2001; 357: 1738-42.
17. Wu JC, Chan FK, Wong SK, Lee YT, Leung WK, Sung JJ. Effect of *Helicobacter pylori* eradication on oesophageal acid exposure in patients with reflux oesophagitis. *Aliment Pharmacol Ther* 2002: 16545-52.

18. Moayyedi P, Feltbower R, Brown J, *et al.* Effect of population screening and treatment for *H. pylori* on dyspepsia and quality of life in the community: a randomised controlled trial. Leeds HELP Study Group. *Lancet* 2000; 13: 1665-9.
19. Chow WH, *et al.* An inverse relation between cagA+ strains of *H. pylori* infection and risk of oesophageal and gastric cardia adenocarcinoma. *Cancer Res* 1998; 15: 588-90.
20. Ye W, *et al. Helicobacter pylori* infection and gastric atrophy: risk of adenocarcinoma and squamous-cell carcinoma of the esophagus and adenocarcinoma of the gastric cardia. *J Natl Cancer Inst* 2004; 3: 388-96.
21. Wu AH, *et al.* Role of *H. pylori* CagA+ strains and risk of adenocarcinoma of the stomach and esophagus. *Int J Cancer* 2003; 1: 815-21.
22. Malfertheiner P, Peitz U, Treiber G. What constitutes failure for *H. pylori* eradication therapy? *Can J Gastroenterol* 2003; 17: 53-7.
23. Gisbert J, Calvet X, Bujanda L, *et al.* "Rescue" therapy with rifabutin after multiple *Helicobacter pylori* treatment failures. *Helicobacter* 2003; 8: 90-4.

The gastroenterologist looks at AIDS

Joep F.W.M. Bartelsman

Academic Medical Center of the University of Amsterdam, Amsterdam, The Netherlands

Gastrointestinal manifestations, mainly caused by opportunistic infections and tumors, are common in patients infected with the human immunodeficiency virus (HIV).

Oesophageal symptoms, chronic diarrhea and anorectal symptoms are the most frequent manifestations.

Endoscopy and endoscopic biopsy are often needed for accurate diagnosis.

This review will focus on the diagnosis and treatment of the most frequent gastrointestinal complications of HIV infections, which will be discussed site by site.

Oesophagus

Dysphagia and odynophagia occur in about 30% of AIDS patients [1].

Candidiasis, cytomegalovirus, herpes simplex, aphtous or idiopathic ulcers and Kaposi's sarcoma are the most common causes.

Biopsies from oesophageal ulcers should include both the ulcer base (where cytomegalovirus inclusions can be found) and the margins (for herpes simplex).

Acute primary HIV-oesophagitis

Oesophagitis can be diagnosed as part of the acute retroviral syndrome or can be the only manifestation of this acute infection [2]. We reported a case of oesophagitis with multiple small shallow ulcerations in a patient who presented with fever, diarrhea, odynophagia and a skin rash [3]. HIV-1 p24 antigen could be shown in the blood on the day of admission. Seroconversion for HIV-1 antibodies took place two weeks later.

Acute HIV-oesophagits can probably be caused by HIV itself. Also transient oesophageal candidiasis can be a complication of acute HIV-infection [4].

Symptoms of HIV primary infection start usually 10-21 days before seroconversion.

Acute primary HIV-oesophagitis heals spontaneously within a week without any therapy.

Candidiasis

The prevalence of *Candida* oesophagitis in AIDS patients with oesophageal symptoms is approximately 50% [5].

Candidiasis usually presents with dysphagia and/or odynophagia.

The positive predictive value of the combination of oropharyngeal candidiasis and oesophageal symptoms for *candida* oesophagitis ranges from 71% to 100% [6].

Oesophageal candidiasis in a immunocompetent patient appears at endoscopy as adherent plaques that may be focal and discrete or confluent.

In AIDS patients colonization becomes more widespread and may be followed by epithelial or deeper invasion into the mucosa and submucosa [7].

Ulcers can occur, but have more often a viral cause (cytomegalovirus or herpes).

Patients with oesophageal candidiasis cannot be treated sufficiently with topical therapy and need a systemic oral azole as the treatment of choice [8].

Compared with ketoconazole, fluconazole has a better safety profile and is better absorbed.

In a prospective study significantly higher rates of endoscopic and symptomatic healing were shown in patients receiving fluconazole as opposed to ketoconazole [9].

Acute treatment of candidiasis episodes is preferred. Recurrences are frequent after successful eradication, but long-term prophylaxis carries the risk of drug-resistant infections.

Other less frequent fungal infections of the oesophagus are those with *Torulopsis glabrata, Histoplasma capsulatum* and *Aspergillus*.

Cytomegalovirus

Cytomegalovirus (CMV) is the most common viral infection of the oesophagus in patients with AIDS. CMV oesophagitis usually presents with dysphagia, severe odynophagia or constant substernal pain.

Endoscopy usually shows solitary or multiple sharply demarcated ulcerations. Ulcers are usually greater than 1 cm in size and are mainly located in the middle or distal third of the oesophagus [10].

The diagnosis depends on the changes detected in endoscopic biopsies. The demonstration of cytomegalic cells on hematoxylin and eosin stained specimens has been considered the gold standard for the diagnosis of CMV oesophagitis [11].

The diagnostic value of biopsy specimen cultures is controversial. A positive culture result does not correlate well with CMV disease and can also be found in biopsies from normal mucosa [12].

CMV responds to either ganciclovir, foscarnet or cidofovir. Ganciclovir is associated mainly with hematological toxicity, while foscarnet and cidofovir are nephrotoxic [13].

In a prospective randomized trial both foscarnet and ganciclovir achieved good clinical response rates: 83% foscarnet-treated and 85% ganciclovir-treated patients showed response clinically and endoscopicaly, but most patients developed further evidence of CMV disease during follow-up [14].

Herpes Simplex Virus

In a immunocompetent host Herpes simplex virus (HSV) oesophagitis may occur as a self-limited acute illness, but in advanced stages of AIDS HSV causes a chronic ulcerated oesophagitis [15].

The major symptoms are dysphagia, odynophagia, chest pain and fever.

The endoscopic picture is variable: in the early phase small rounded vesicles in the mid to distal oesophagus can be seen, but more often small, discrete, punched-out ulcers with normal surrounding mucosa.

In severe cases the ulcers coalesce and denudation of the entire squamous mucosa ensues [7].

Brushings and biopsies must be taken from the margins of the ulcers. Cultures of biopsy specimens are the most sensitive.

HSV oesophagitis responds quickly to aciclovir, but maintenance therapy may be indicated in patients with recurrent disease.

Idiopathic oesophageal (aphthous) ulcers

This diagnosis is made in AIDS patients with oesophageal ulcers without any identifiable cause after careful pathologic examination of biopsy specimens.

In a study of 100 consecutive HIV infected patients with oesophageal ulcerations a diagnosis of idiopathic aphthous ulcer was made in 40%, almost as frequent as the most common cause ulcers, caused by CMV infection [16].

Severe odynophagia, chest pain and weight loss are the main symptoms.

Barium radiography and endoscopy show large, undermined ulcers, located in the mid to distal oesophagus, that can be complicated by fistula, mucosal bridging and perforation.

Prednison (orally, intravenously, or injected in the lesions) results in quick pain relief and ulcer healing in the majority of patients, but relapse occurs after discontinuation of therapy.

Thalidomide is also a very effective drug as treatment of refractory idiopathic aphthous ulceration. In an Australian study 19 of 20 patients had a dramatic response to thalidomide therapy [17].

Stomach

The stomach is not often involved as a consequence of HIV infection [18].

We diagnosed Kaposi's sarcoma (KS) in the stomach in 36 of 65 patients with gastrointestinal KS, mostly without any gastric symptoms *(figures 1 and 2)*. Also AIDS related lymphoma can occur in the stomach and present as a gastric ulcer. Occasionally CMV gastritis can cause erosions or ulcers [19].

Mycobacterium avium complex (MAC) and cryptosporidiosis also occur in the stomach.

Gastric involvement in AIDS related cryptosporidiosis can often be found, if biopsies are taken, but clear correlation between gastric involvement and related clinical and pathological features was observed [20].

Small intestine

Diarrhea is a common gastrointestinal symptom of AIDS, affecting 50-90% of patients [21].

Among 1,933 patients of the Swiss HIV Cohort Study 560 diarrheal episodes were evaluated: 212 episodes of acute diarrhea and 348 of chronic diarrhea [22]. The risk to develop diarrhea was significantly higher for homosexual men, patients with a history of opportunistic complications and patients taking antiretroviral therapy.

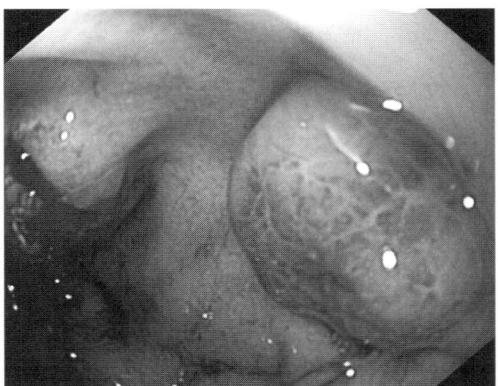 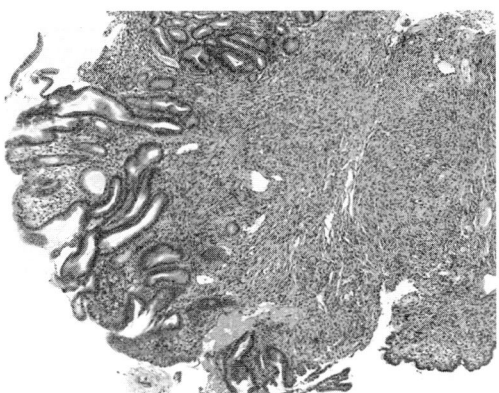

Figure 1. Stomach. Kaposi's sarcoma.

Figure 2. Stomach. Kaposi's sarcoma. Endoscopic biopsy specimen, showing submucosal tumor with spindled cells with irregular, slit-like luminal spaces and extravasated red cells.

Causes of AIDS diarrhea include bacteria (MAI, *Clostridium difficile*, *Salmonella*, *Shigella* and *Campylobacter jejuni*) viruses (CMV, HSV, possibly HIV) and protozoa (*Cryptosporidium parvum*, *Isospora belli*, *Enterocytozoon bieneusi*, *Septata intestinalis*, *Cyclospora spp*, *Entamoeba histolytica* and *Giardia lamblia*).

By examinations of stools, duodenal, jejunal and rectal biopsy specimens and duodenal aspirate for bacterial, protozoal and viral pathogens a specific cause of diarrhea can be found in the majority of patients. In a prospective study of 155 patients with AIDS and chronic diarrhea, 83% had at least one potential pathogen [23]. Stool analysis identified the most pathogens (47%).

In a prospective study in patients with HIV and chronic diarrhea for which no cause could be found 39 of 155 patients were recruited [24].

On follow-up a possible cause of diarrhea was identified in eight. In 17 of the remaining 31, the diarrhea resolved completely in a mean of seven months from its onset.

Protozoal infections

- ***Cryptosporidium parvum*** is one of the main causes of diarrhea in HIV infected patients and is more common in male homosexuals and children [25]. Oral-anal contact is propably a way of transmission.

In patients with low CD4 counts cryptosporidiosis can cause a chronic devastating illness with severe dehydration, electrolyte imbalance and wasting.

The infection can be diagnosed by showing oocysts with stool examination by the modified acid-fast stain and microscopy or by enzyme-linked immunosorbent assays (ELISAs).

Endoscopically the small bowel mucosa is erythematous and granular. Biopsies show irregular, shortened and fused villi [26].

Cryptosporidia are small round basophilic bodies on the surface of the intestinal absorptive cells.

Supportive therapy and rehydration are the most important treatment options.

Antisecretory drugs such as octreotide and vapreotide have had mixed results [27].

Many drugs have been tried to eradicate *cryptosporium*, the most promising are paromomycine and nitazoxanide [28, 29].

At the moment the most effective eradication is improvement of immunodeficiency by the treatment of the HIV infection itself.

- **Microsporidiosis** is found in about 30% of AIDS patients with chronic diarrhea and can cause malabsorpion and wasting [30].

The organisms are very small and round and located at the apical cytoplasm of the enterocytes in the villi. In the past the diagnosis could only be made by electron microscopy of jejunal biopsies, but nowadays, by better staining methods, a light microscopic diagnosis of biopsy specimens, jejunal aspirates and stool samples is possible [31].

There are several species of *Microspora*: 90% of the infections in AIDS patients are caused by *Enterocytozoon bieneusi*.

Encephalitozoon intestinalis (or *Septata intestinalis*) is not only present in the enterocytes, but also in macrophages in the *lamina propria* and can cause systemic infection.

This species, along with CMV, cryptosporidia and atypical mycobacteria can play a role in AIDS-related cholangitis [32].

Encephalitozoon can usually be effectively treated with albendazole [33].

Therapeutic approaches for *E. bieneusi* are still difficult

Albendazole can give symptomatic improvement but doesn't eradicate *E. bieneusi* [34].

- **Isospora belli** is, especially in developing countries, a frequent cause of chronic diarrhea in AIDS patients. Isosporiasis can easily be detected in the stool: the oocysts are much larger than those of other coccidian protozoans.

Endoscopic biopsy can show organisms within vacuoles in enterocytes.

Isosporiasis can be treated with many antibiotics. Trimethoprim-sulfamethoxazole is the treatment of choice. Long-term treatment is often necessary, because of the high recurrence rate.

- ***Cyclospora cayetanensis*** is another protozoan, causing chronic diarrhea in immunocompromized patients in tropical countries. Diagnosis is made by stool examination. Like in isosporiasis, there is a good response to treatment with trimethoprim-sulfamethoxazole with a high recurrence rate [35].

- ***Giardia lamblia*** can cause diarrhea in AIDS patients, especially in male homosexuals. Infection takes place *via* contaminated water or by oral-anal contact. Giardiasis responds to therapy with metronidazole or tinidazole.

Bacterial infections

Mycobacterium avium complex (MAC) is the most common systemic bacterial infection in patients with AIDS. MAC causes a disseminated infection with involvement of lymph nodes, liver, spleen, and gut, most often the small bowel.

Infected patients have very low CD4 counts (< 50), abdominal pain, anorexia, fever and weight loss.

The duodenum mucosa shows white or yellow patches and enlarged villi, microscopically the *lamina propria* contains macrophages packed with organisms, simulating Whipple's disease, but acid-fast staining is negative in Whipple's disease and strongly positive in MAC enteritis [36].

Disseminated MAC infection is a frequent cause of death among HIV patients [37].

Early diagnosis and treatment of MAC infection is important. Symptomatic improvement, improved survival and, after prolonged treatment, eradication of MAC can be reached only by a combination of three or four drugs, for example clarithromycin, ethambutol and rifabutin [38].

Patients with CD4 counts < 50 cells/micro L should receive MAC prophylaxis, preferable with clarithromycin or azithromycin [39].

In patients responding to highly active antiretroviral therapy (HAART) maintenance therapy against MAC can be discontinued [40].

In developing countries tuberculosis is a common HIV-related opportunistic infection and an important cause of death. It is estimated that in 1999 HIV-related tuberculosis reached 1,000,000 cases and caused 30% of the 2,500,000 AIDS-related deaths [39].

M. tuberculosis can infect the gut, mostly the small bowel and ileocoecal area, complicated by ileum obstruction, perforation or fistulas. In contrast to the diffuse MAC infection, tuberculosis generally causes segemental and granulomatous inflammation and can occur early in HIV infection.

Colon

Colonoscopy and colonic biopsy is an effective method of identifying the cause of diarrhea in AIDS patients, when examination of the stool is negative. CMV and MAC are the most common infections found. Also severe pseudomembranous colitis can occur in AIDS, requiring treatment for *Clostridium difficile*.

In addition to opportunistic causes also common bacterial pathogens can be associated with severe diarrhea, particularly in male homosexual AIDS patients.

Cytomegalovirus

Cytomegalovirus (CMV), the most important cause of chronic colitis in patients with AIDS, usually occurs after the CD4 cells have fallen below 100/mm3. Patients present with chronic or intermittent diarrhea, rectal blood loss, fever and malaise.

Complications of CMV infection are hemorrhage, perforation obstruction and toxic megacolon.

Those complications of CMV infections are responsible for one third of all surgery in AIDS patients and for about 50% of cases with severe lower gastrointestinal bleeding [41, 42].

The endoscopic picture is variable. In some patients the mucosa appears granular and friable with areas of oedema and erythema, caused by mucosal and sumucosal hemorrhage. In other patients colonoscopy shows solitary or multiple deep sharply demarcated ulcerations.

Also pseudomembranous colitis can be caused by CMV alone [43].

The right and transverse colon are more often involved than the left colon, so complete colonoscopy is sometimes needed to establish the diagnosis.

Endoscopic biopsies should preferentially be taken from the center of an ulcer.

Charasteristic findings of CMV infection are basophilic intranuclear inclusions surrounded by a halo.

This results in the so-called owl's eye appearance.

Patients with CMV colitis are treated for 2-3 weeks with ganciclovir or foscarnet [13, 14]. In case of only partial response prolonged treatment is needed.

Other viruses

Non-CMV enteric viral infections are likely to account for a significant proportion of pathogen-negative diarrhea in HIV patients.

Rotavirus, adenovirus and coxsackie virus have been implicated as causative agents.

In a prospective study the association of enteric viruses with symptoms was investigated in 377 HIV-infected patients with diarrhea [44].

A 15,9% prevalence of non-CMV enteric viral infections was found: adenovirus 7,2%, rotavirus 2,4%, coronavirus 2,9% and small round structured viruses (SRSV) in 1,3%.

Enteric viral infections were found to be significantly associated with acute diarrhea. The presence of adenovirus colitis was significantly more likely to be associated with chronic diarrhea than adenovirus isolated from stool alone.

The causal role of adenovirus in the pathogenesis of diarrhea is questionable, because many infected patients remain asymptomatic.

Bacterial infections

Persistent *Salmonella* (in particular *S. typhimurium*), *Shigella* and *Campylobacter* infections are frequently decribed in immunosuppressed patients [45].

Shigella and *Campylobacter* can be transmitted by ingestion of contaminated food, but also venereally. In AIDS patients there is a high risk of bacteremia and a long-term asymptomatic carrier state, probably because of inadequate T-cell function.

Diagnosis is made by stool culture, but also by blood culture.

The treatment of bacterial pathogens in patients with AIDS is similar to the therapy in immunocompetent patients, but antibiotic treatment is always recommended in patients with AIDS, to treat and prevent invasive disease.

Also *Clostridium difficile* associated pseudomembranous colitis is common in patients with AIDS, probably as a consequence of antibiotic agents to treat or prevent opportunistic infections.

C. difficile toxin detection is the preferred method of diagnosis.

Colitis by *C. difficile* responds rapidly to treatment with oral vancomycine or metronidazole, but relapses occur often after discontinuation of treatment.

Pseudomembranous colitis can als be caused by CMV in the absence of *C. difficile* [43].

Idiopathic colitis

Idiopathic colitis with mucosal inflammation and ulcerations has been decribed in patients with AIDS.

Gopal decribed eight cases with HIV infection, who had diarrhea for more than four weeks and colitis with ulcerations at endoscopy [46]. In all cases no specific pathogen could be detected despite extensive evaluation. The patients were treated with prednisone. The diarrhea completely resolved in three and improved in five patients.

After a minimum follow-up of eight months only in one patient an enteric pathogen was found.

Anorectum

Male homosexuals with AIDS frequently develop anorectal problems.

Herpes simplex virus (HSV) is the most common cause of perianal ulcers and proctitis.

Tenesmus, fever, and severe anal and rectal pain are the major complaints.

In a study of 272 hospitalized AIDS patients, perianal ulcers were found in 23 (9%).

The presence of HSV DNA was shown in 22 of the 23 patients [47].

Acyclovir is the treatment of choice. Long-term therapy is often indicated.

Anorectal ulcers can also be caused by CMV and *Histoplasma capsulatum* [48].

Ideopathic anal ulcers resemble, histologically, those in the oesophagus.

These occur typically when the CD4 count is less than 200.

Surgery is often indicated [49].

Injections with corticosteroids into the ulcer base or margins diminishes the pain, associated with the lesion [50]. Also thalidomide may play a role.

HIV-related tumors

Before the introduction of highly active antiretroviral therapy (HAART) malignancies accounted for less than 10% of all deaths among HIV-infected patients. As a result of decreased occurrence of opportunistic infections and the possible oncogenic role of HIV itself this figure has increased.

In a survey in all French hospitals of a total of 964 deaths, 269 (28%) were attributable to malignancies [51]. AIDS-related malignancies were the underlying cause of 149 deaths (15%), non-AIDS-related malignancies were the cause of death in 13%.

The main HIV-related malignancies involving the gastrointestinal tract are Kaposi's sarcoma (KS), non-Hodgkin lymphoma (NHL) and anal squamous carcinoma.

The current incidence of KS among patients with HIV is less than 10% of the incidence reported in 1994 and also the incidence of NHL is decreased since the introduction of HAART [52, 53].

However, anal cancer is an increasing problem among HIV-infected persons.

Kaposi's sarcoma

Kaposi's sarcoma (KS) is frequently found in the gut of patients with cutaneous involvement.

Widely reported risk factors for KS include acquisition of HIV *via* homosexual contact and advanced immunosuppression [53]. Moore and Chang found herpesviruslike DNA sequences in KS tissue obtained from a patient with AIDS [54]. This virus was named *human herpesvirus 8* (HHV-8).

Postmortem studies show that the majority of patients with cutaneous KS have gut involvement and that lesions in the gastrointestinal tract may occur in the absence of any skin lesion.

KS may develop in any part of the gastrointestinal tract and is mostly asymptomatic. Extensive involvement may lead to thickening of the intestinal wall, intestinal obstruction and diarrhea.

Serious gastrointestinal bleeding is uncommon.

In our hospital we diagnosed one or more KS lesions in the gastrointestinal tract in 65 out of 225 admitted AIDS patients: in the oropharynx in 35, oesophagus in 17, stomach in 36, duodenum in 21, small intestine in 13, colon and rectum in 27 patients.

The endoscopic appearance of KS in the gut is variable: small flat red or violet lesions, sessile red polyps, sometimes with central ulceration or larger tumors.

Because most KS lesions are submucosal, endoscopic biopsies are often false-negative.

Histologically KS is characterized by a proliferation of dilated capillaries with atypical endothelial cells, spindle cells, extravasation of erythrocytes and hemosiderin and often eosinophilic round cytoplasmic globules [55].

HAART is not only associated with a decreased number of KS cases, but also with a regression of existing KS.

Other treatment options are drugs targeting at HHV-8, and the processes of angiogenesis and cellular differentiation [56].

AIDS-related non-Hodgkin's lymphoma (NHL)

HIV-associated NHL's are most common in the small intestine and colon [55]. At least 95% are B-cell lymphomas. EBV expression is found in the majority of these lymphomas.

In the gastrointestinal tract NHL usually presents with bleeding, abdominal pain or obstruction.

Endoscopically solitary or multiple nodular lesions, sometimes with ulcerations can be seen.

In the era before HAART dose-intense combination regimens were abandoned because of difficulties in tolerating aggressive chemotherapy in the presence of underlying immunosuppression, but with improvements in supportive care and more effective anti-retroviral therapies nowadays the chemotherapeutic approaches are similar to those used in the non-HIV infected NHL patients [57].

Anal squamous carcinoma

Anal condylomata with dysplasia or *in situ* carcinoma and anal squamous carcinomas are common in male homosexuals, particularly male homosexuals with AIDS [55].

Since the introduction of HAART the incidence of anal cancer in patients with HIV is increased, probably by a significant decrease in mortality and prolonged survival.

Despite the evidence that HIV infection increases the likelihood of human papillomavirus (HPV) infection and the subsequent development of high-grade anal intraepithelial neoplasia, it is unclear whether HIV infection itself has a direct effect on the development of anal cancer [58].

Anal Pap testing of HIV-positive homosexual men has been suggested as a cost-effective means of preventing invasive cancer [59].

The majority of patients with HPV-induced anal carcinoma can be cured by combination treatment with external-beam radiotherapy and chemotherapy.

References

1. Connolly GM, Hawkins D, Harcourt-Webster JN, Parsons PA, Husain OA, Gazzard BG. Oesophageal symptoms, their causes, treatment, and prognosis in patients with a. The acquired immunodeficiency syndrome. *Gut* 1989; 30: 1033-9.
2. Schmassmann-Suhijar D, Schmassmann A, Aphtous esophagitis as an atypical manifestation of a primary HIV-infection. *Dtsc Med Wochenschr* 2001; 126: 1136-8.
3. Bartelsman JFWM, Lange JM, van Leeuwen R, van den Tweel JG, Tytgat GN. Acute primary HIV-esophagitis. *Endoscopy* 1990; 22: 184-5.

4. Pena JM, Martinez-Lopez MA, Arnalich F, Barbado FJ, Vazquez JJ. Esophageal candidiasis associated with acute infection due to human immunodeficiency virus: case report and review. *Rev Infect Dis* 1991; 13: 872-5.
5. Bonacini M, Young T, Laine L. The causes of esophageal symptoms in human immunodeficiency virus infection. A prospective study of 110 patients. *Arch Intern Med* 1991; 11: 1567-71.
6. Connolly GM, Forbes A, Gleeson JA, Gazzard BG.Investigation of upper gastrointestinal symptoms in patients with AIDS. *AIDS* 1989; 3: 453-6.
7. Baehr PH, McDonald GB. Esophageal infections: Risk factors, presentation, diagnosis and treatment. *Gastroenterology* 1994; 106: 509-32.
8. Powderly WG, Gallant JE, Ghannoum MA, Mayer KH, Navarro EE, Perfect JR. Oropharyngela candidiasis in patients with HIV: suggested guidelines for therapy. *AIDS Res Hum Retroviruses* 1999; 15: 1619-23.
9. Laine L,Dretler RH, Conteas CN, Tuazon C,Koster FM, Sattler F, Squires K, Islam MZ. Fluconazole compared with ketoconazole for the treatment of candida esophagitis in AIDS. *Ann Intern Med* 1992; 117: 655-60.
10. Wilcox CM, Straub RF, Schwartz DA. Prospective endoscopic characterization of cytomegalovirus esophagitis in AIDS. *Gastrointest Endosc* 1994; 40: 481-4.
11. Wilcox CM, Diehl DL, Cello JP, Margaretten W, Jacobson MA. Cytomegalovirus esophagitis in patients with AIDS. A clinical, endoscopic and pathologic correlation. *Ann Inern Med* 1990; 113: 589-93.
12. Goodgame RW, Genta RM, Estrada R, Demmler G, Buffone G. Frequency of positive tests for cytomegalovirus in AIDS patients: endoscopic lesions compared with normal mucosa. *Am J Gastroenterol* 1993; 88: 338-43.
13. Cheung TW, Teich SA. Cytomegalovirus infection in patients with HIV infection. *Mt Sinai J Med* 1999; 66: 113-24.
14. Blanshard C, Benhamou Y, Dohin E, Lernestedt JO, Gazzard BG, Katlama C. Treatment of AIDS-associated cytomegalovirus infection with foscarnet and ganciclovir: a randomized comparison. *J Infect Dis* 1995; 172: 622-8.
15. Genereau T, Lortholary O, Bouchaud O, Lacassin F, Vinceneux P, De Truchis P, *et al.* Herpes simplex esophagitis in patients with AIDS: report of 34 cases. The Cooperative Study Group on Herpetic Esophagitis in HIV infection. *Vlin Infect Dis* 1996; 22: 926-31.
16. Wilcox CM, Schwartz DA, Scott Clark W. Esopageal ulceration in Human Immunodeficiency Virus infection. *Ann Intern Med* 1995; 123: 143-9.
17. Paterson DL, Georghiou PR, Allworth AM, Kemp RJ. Thalidomide as treatment of refractory aphthous ulceration related to human immunodeficiency virus infection. *Clin Infect Dis* 1995; 20: 250-4.
18. Corley DA, Cello JP, Koch J. Evaluation of upper gastrointestinal tract symptoms in patients infected with HIV. *Am J Gastroenterol* 1999; 94: 2890-6.
19. Vachon GC, Brown BS, Kim C,Chessin LN.CMV gastric ulcer as the presenting manifestation of AIDS. *Am J Gastroenterol* 1995; 90: 319-21.
20. Rossi P, Rivasi F, Codeluppi M, Catania A, Tamburrini A, Righi E, *et al.* Gastric involvement in AIDS associated cryptosporidiosis. *Gut* 1998; 43: 476-7.
21. Chui DW, Owen RL. AIDS and the gut. *J Gastroenterol Hepatol* 1994; 9: 291-303.
22. Weber R, Ledergerber B, Zbinden R, Altwegg M, Pfyffer GE, Spycher MA, *et al.* Enteric infections and diarrhea in Human Immunodeficiency Virus-infected persons. Prospective community-based cohort stydy. *Arch Intern Med* 1999; 159: 1473-7.
23. Blanshard C, Francis N, Gazzard BG. Investigation of chronic diarrhea in acquired immunodeficiency syndrome. A prospective study of 155 patients. *Gut* 1996; 39: 824-32.
24. Blanshard C, Gazzard BG. Natural history and prognosis of diarrhea of unknown cause in patients with acquired immunodeficiency syndrome (AIDS). *Gut* 1995; 36: 283-6.

25. Navin TR, Hardy AM. Cryptosporidiosis in patients with AIDS. *J Infect Dis* 1987; 11: 150.
26. Clayton F, Heller T, Kotler DP. Variation in the enteric distribution of cryptosporidia in acquired immunodeficiency syndrome. *Am J Clin Pathol* 1994; 102: 420-5.
27. Girard PM, Goldschmidt E, Vittecoq D, Massip P, Gastiaburu J, Meyohas MC, et al. Vapreotide, a somatostatin analogue, in cryptosporidiosis and other AIDS-related diarroeal diseases. *AIDS* 1992; 6: 715-8.
28. Chappell CL, Okhuysen PC. Cryptosporidiosis. *Curr Opin Infect Dis* 2002; 15: 523-7.
29. Rossignol JF, Hidalgo H, Feregrino M, Higuera F, Gomez WH, Romero JL, et al. A double-"blind" placebo-controlled study of nitazoxanide in the treatmen of cryptosporidial diarrhoea in AIDS patients in Mexico. *Trans R Soc Trop Med Hyg* 1998; 92: 663-6.
30. Eeftinck Schattenkerk JK, van Gool T, van Ketel RJ, Bartelsman JF, Kuiken CL, Terpstra WJ, et al. Clinical significance of small-intestinal microsporidiosis in HIV-1-infected individuals. *Lancet* 1991; 337: 895-8.
31. van Gool T, Snijders F, Reiss P, Eeftinck Schattenkerk JK, van den Bergh Weerman MA, Bartelsman JF, et al. Diagnosis of intestinal and disseminated microsporidial infections in patients with HIV by a new rapid fluorescence technique. *J Clin Pathol* 1993; 46: 694-9.
32. Lippert U, Schottelius J, Manegold C. Disseminated microsporidiosis (Encephalitozoon intestinalis) in a patient with HIV infection. *Dtsch Med Wochenschr* 2003; 128: 1769-72.
33. Gross U. Treatment of microsporidiosis including albendazole. *Parasitol Res* 2003; 90: S14-8.
34. Dieterich DT, Lew EA, Kotler DP, Poles MA, Orenstein JM. Treatment with albendazole for intestinal disease due to Enterocytozoon bieneusi in patients with AIDS. *J Infect Dis* 1994; 169: 178-83.
35. Pape JW, Verdier RI, Boncy M, Boncy J, Johnson WD Jr. Cyclospora infection in adults infected with HIV. Clinical manifestations, treatment and prophylaxis. *Ann Intern Med* 1994; 121: 654-7.
36. Cappell MS, Philogene C. The endoscopic appearance of severe intestinal Mycobacterium avium complex infection as a coarsely granular mucosa due to massive infiltration and expansion of intestinal villi without mucosal exudation. *J Clin Gastroenterol* 1995; 21: 323-6.
37. Bellamy R, Sangeetha S, Paton NI. Causes of death among patients with HIV in Singnapore from 1985 to 2001: results from the Singapore HIV Observational Cohort Study (SHOCS). *HIV Med* 2004; 5: 289-95.
38. Benson CA, Williams PL, Currier JS, Holland F, Mahon LF, MacGregor, et al. A prospective, randomized trial examining the efficacy and safety of clarithromycin in combination with ethambutol, rifabutin or both for the treatment of disseminated Mycobacterium avium complex disease in persons with acquired immunodeficiency syndrome. *Clin Infect Dis* 2003; 37: 1234-43.
39. Pozniak A. Mycobacterial disease and HIV. *J HIV Ther* 2002; 7: 13-6.
40. Rossi M, Flepp M, Telenti A, Schiffer V, Egloff N, Bucher H, et al. Disseminated M. Avium complex infection in the Swiss HIV Cohort Study: declining incidence, improved prognosis and discontinuation of maintenance therapy. *Swiss Med Wkly* 2001; 131: 471-7.
41. Chalasani N, Wilcox CM. Etiology and outcome of lower gastrointestinal bleeding in patients with AIDS. *Am J Gastroenterol* 1998; 93: 175-8.
42. Ferguson CM. Surgical complications of human immune deficiency virus infection. *Am Surg* 1988; 54: 4-9.
43. Olofinlade O, Chiang C. Cytomegalovirus infection as a cause of pseudomembranous colitis: a report of four cases. *J Clin Gastroenterol* 2001; 32: 82-4.
44. Thomas PD, Pollok RCG, Gazzard BG. Enteric viral infections as a cause of diarrhea in the acquired immunodeficiency syndrome. *HIV Med* 1999; 1: 19-24.
45. Lew EA, Poles MA, Dieterich DT. Diarrheal diseases associated with HIV infection. *Gastroenterol Clin North Am* 1997; 26: 259-90.
46. Gopal DV, Hassaram S, Marcon NE, Kandel G. Idiopathic colonic inflammation in AIDS: an open trial of prednisone. *Am J Gastroenterol* 1997; 92: 2237-40.

47. Nascimento MC, Pannuti CS, Nascimento CM, Sumita LM, Eluf-Neto J. Prevalence and risk factors associated with perianal ulcer in advanced acquired immunodeficiency syndrome. *Int J Infect Dis* 2002; 6: 253-8.
48. Winburn GB, Yeh KA. Severe anal ulceration secondary to Histoplasma capsulatum in a patient with HIV disease. *Am Surg* 1999; 65: 321-2.
49. Nadal SR, Manzione CR, Horta SH, Galvao V. Management of idiopathic ulcer of the anal canal by excision in HIV-positive patients. *Dis Colon Rectum* 1999; 42: 598-601.
50. Paré AA, Gottesman L. Anorectal diseases. *Gastroenterol Clin North Am* 1997; 26: 367-76.
51. Bonnet F, Lewden C, May T, Heripret L, Jougla E, Bevilacqua S, *et al*. Malignancy-related causes of death in human immunodeficiency virus-infected patients in the era of highly active antiretroviral therapy. *Cancer* 2004; 101; 317-24.
52. Gates AE, Kaplan LD. AIDS malignancies in the era of highly active antiretroviral therapy. *Oncology (Huntingt)* 2002; 16: 657-65.
53. Mocroft A, Kirk O, Clumeck N, Gargalianos-Kakolyris P,Trocha H, Chentsova N, *et al*. The changing pattern of Kaposi's sarcoma in patients with HIV, 1994-2003. The EuroSIDA Study. *Cancer* 2004; 100: 2644-54.
54. Moore PS, Chang Y. Detection of herpesvirus-like DNA sequences in Kaposi's sarcoma in patients with and without HIV infection. *N Eng J Med* 1995; 332: 1181-5.
55. Clayton F, Clayton CH. Gastrointestinal pathology in HIV-infected patients. *Gastroenterol Clin North Am* 1997; 26: 191-240.
56. Dezube BJ, Pantanowitz L, Aboulafia DM. Management of AIDS-related Kaposi's sarcoma:advances in target discovery and treatment. *AIDS Read* 2004; 14: 236-8.
57. Stebbing J, Marvin V, Bower M. The evidence-based treatment of AIDS-related non-Hodgkin's lymphoma. *Cancer Treat Rev* 2004; 30: 249-53.
58. Ryan DP, Compton CC,Mayer RJ. Carcinoma of the anal canal. *N Eng J Med* 2000; 342: 792-800.
59. Berry JM, Palefsky JM, Welton ML. Anal cancer and its precursors in HIV-positive patients: perspectives and management. *Surg Oncol Clin North Am* 2004; 13: 355-73.

Modern management of echinococcosis

Hans G. Schipper

Department of Internal Medicine, Division of Infectious Diseases, Tropical Medicine and AIDS, Academic Medical Center, Amsterdam, The Netherlands

Echinococcosis is a zoonosis transmitted by dogs in livestock-raising areas and accidentally affects man. Worldwide, infection with the larval stage of the dog tapeworm *Echinococcus granulosus* occurs most frequently. This relatively benign parasitic disease is characterised by slowly growing cysts, most commonly in the liver, less frequently in lungs and rarely elsewhere in the body. Developing countries with poor hygiene where sheep and cattle are raised, are high-risk areas for acquiring cystic echinococcosis.

Infection with the larvae of the fox tapeworm *Echinococcus multilocularis* occurs in fewer areas. *Echinococcus multilocularis* causes slowly progressive liver necrosis which tends to metastasise and behave like a malignant disease. Colder climates, mountain and forest areas housing foxes are the primary risk areas for acquiring alveolar echinococcosis. Infection with *Echinococcus vogeli* (jaguar tapeworm) and *Echinococcus oligarthrus* (puma tapeworm) is rare and occurs only in South America.

This paper will focus on cystic echinococcosis of the liver, the most relevant type of echinococcosis in the world.

Pathogenesis and etiology

Dogs are the definite host of *Echinococcus granulosus* and harbour the tapeworm in the small intestine. Sheep and cattle are the intermediate host and become feco-orally infected by *Echinococcus* eggs shed into the environment with feces of infected dogs. *Echinococcus* eggs hatch in the intestinal mucosa of the intermediate host and transform into oncospheres which penetrate bowell wall. Through the portal circulation the liver is reached where slowly expanding cysts develop. The cyst wall consists of a double layer, the inner side forms a germinal layer where protoscoleces grow which secrete clear fluid.

This brood capsule may generate daughter cysts by invagination. The intermediate host responds to the presence of the parasitic cyst by surrounding it with fibrous tissue. This complex of parasitic cyst plus fibrous capsule is called *Echinococcus* cyst or hydatid cyst. Life cycle is closed when dogs are infected by viable cyst-containing organs of slaughtered livestock. In the intestine of the dog, protoscoleces develop into adult tapeworms *(figure 1)* [1, 2].

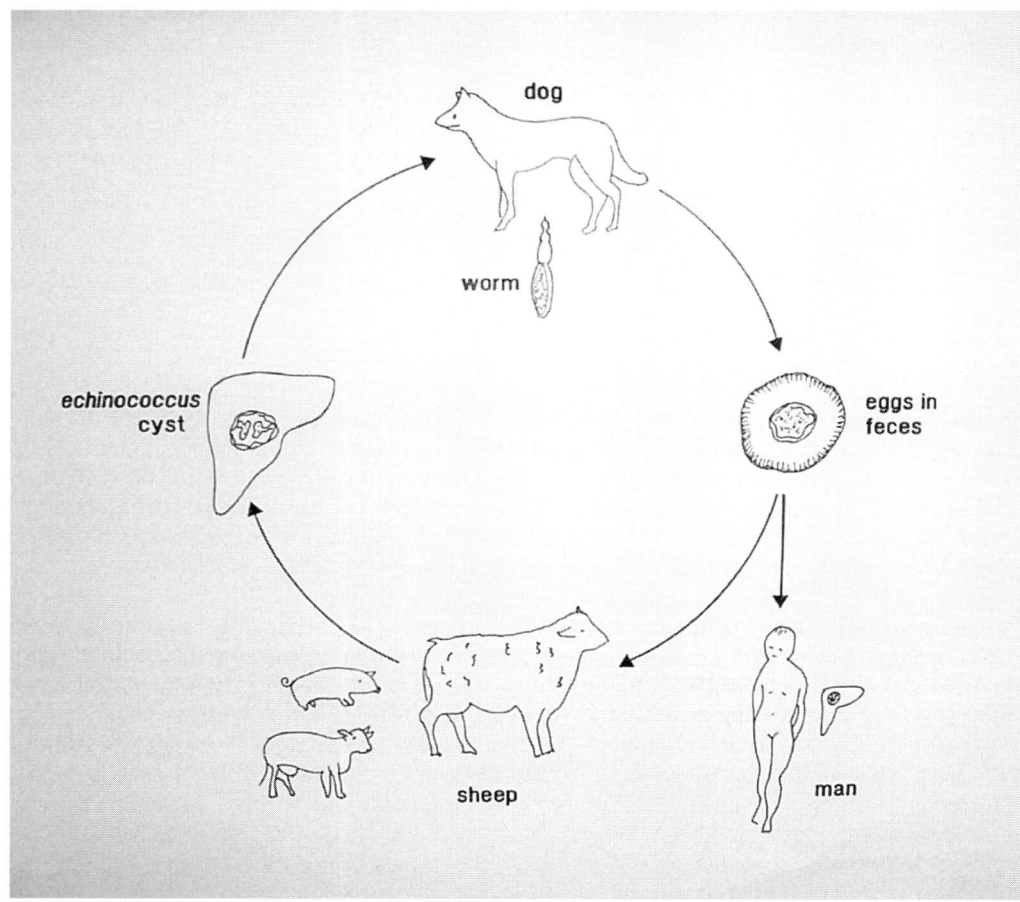

Figure 1. Lifecycle of *Echinococcus granulosus*.

Man is a dead end host and becomes feco-orally infected by *Echinococcus* eggs.

Autochthonic people in endemic areas are the primary risk group, less frequently aid workers and rarely tourists. Children playing with infected dogs may become infected early in life. Due to slowly growth, cysts become usually symptomatic a few years after infection, in adolescence or early adulthood. Infected adults may become symptomatic later in life. However, host immunity may overcome parasitic infection making the *Echinococcus* cyst non-viable without ever becoming symptomatic.

Epidemiology

Echinococcosis is prevalent worldwide. High prevalence is found in parts of Southern and Eastern Europe, former USSR, Middle East, Northern and Eastern Africa, North-western Kenya (Turkana), Southern Sudan, Ethiopia, Eritrea, North-western and Eastern China, South America. Sporadic infections occur in North America, South-western United States, Central America, Northern South America, South Africa, Australia, New Zealand and Northern Europe.

In West European countries where echinococcosis is not endemic, the disease is diagnosed primarily in immigrants from Mediterranean countries such as Morocco, Turkey and the former Yugoslavia. Less frequently in immigrants from Greece, Italy and Spain. An increasing number of patients are diagnosed in asylum seekers from the Middle East and other endemic countries.

Diagnosis

The diagnosis is based on (i) history and geography, (ii) imaging and (iii) serology. Parasitology of cyst content confirms the diagnosis. Most cysts occur in the liver (52-77%), less frequently in lungs (8.5-44%) or elsewhere in the body (15-19%) [3]

Clinical features

Right upper abdominal pain due to the mass effect of the enlarging cyst, is the most characteristic symptom. Pain may be intermittent or continuous and gradually increasing over a long period of time. When located in epigastrio, it is easily mistaken for gastritis, gastric ulcer or cholelithiasis. Malaise, anorexia and abdominal distension are accompanying symptoms. Urticaria, asthma-like symptoms and fever may occur as a response to the *Echinococcus* antigen in cyst fluid. Sometimes patients identify an abdominal mass themselves. Physical examination is frequently insignificant. Most common physical signs are raised right hemi diaphragm, a tender enlarged liver or a palpable liver mass. Laboratory tests are often completely normal. Eosinophilia may be present or slightly elevated alkaline phosphatase or gamma glutamyltransferase.

Complications

Anaphylactic shock, cyst infection and rupture into the biliary tree are the most severe complications.

- **Anaphylactic shock** due to spontaneous or traumatic cyst rupture or during surgery is a rare and severe complication. Patients may die when diagnosis is not recognised, appropriate treatment is not immediately at hand or anaphylaxis is refractory to treatment [4-7].

Seeding of cyst content into the peritoneal cavity is a serious secondary complication of cyst rupture. Viable protoscoleces may develop into new hydatid cysts causing substantial morbidity in the future.

- **Cysts** may become infected following bacteremia or via communicating bile ducts, especially when ERCP has been performed. These patients present with high fever, sepsis syndrome and a tender liver. Like in liver abscess, antibiotics and drainage are the principals of treatment.

- **Rupture** into the biliary tree typically occurs in larger cysts containing multiple daughter cysts. Clinical characteristics are recurrent colic pain, transient obstruction jaundice and fever. Because these symptoms mimic those of obstructing bile stones, the diagnosis intrabiliary rupture is easily overlooked. Treatment is based on cyst drainage, antibiotics and sphincterotomy to remove obstructing membrane fragments from the biliary tree and to lower intrabiliary pressure.

- **Less threatening complications** are related to the mass effect of the cyst and comprise compression of bile ducts and portal or hepatic veins. This may result in obstructive jaundice, post obstructive cholangitis and impaired blood flow of portal and hepatic veins. Treatment is primarily directed on resolution of the mass effect by percutaneous or surgical intervention.

Imaging

Ultrasonography (US) is the preferred diagnostic tool for hepatic hydatid cysts. It is easy available, cost-effective and used for classification and estimation of cyst viability. Gharbi related preoperative US-findings to viability of protoscoleces at surgery and classified five different types. Type 1, univesicular hypodense cyst containing "hydatid sand", is diagnostic for a hydatid cyst, but not without it. Type 2, univesicular hypodense cyst with a double or undulating membrane, and type 3, so-called "mother and daughter" cyst, are highly specific for hydatidosis. Type 4 and type 5 cysts are degenerated cysts. Type 4 cysts show several aspects: detachment of the germinal layer sometimes with a so-called "water Lilly" sign, echogenic content with solidification or a pseudotumor aspect. In addition to these characteristics, type 5 cysts contain cyst wall calcifications. Types 1, 2 and 3 appeared to be viable cysts at postoperative parasitological examination and type 4 and 5 non-viable cysts *(figures 2-5)* [8].

Usually, CT-scan is the next step after US diagnosis has been made. The main purpose is to visualise the relation of the hydatid cyst to the surrounding liver tissue, bile ducts, portal and hepatic veins and its segmental location. MRI is not indicated for routine diagnosis but only when complications are suspected such as transdiaphragmatic extension of the cyst complex into the pleural cavity.

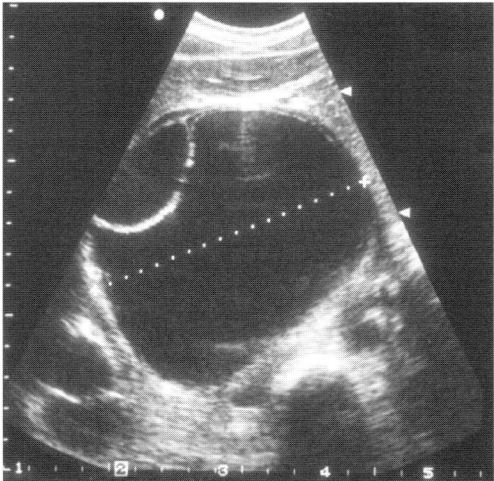

Figure 2. Ultrasound showing univesicular (Gharbi type 2) cyst with "double membrane" and one daughter cyst.

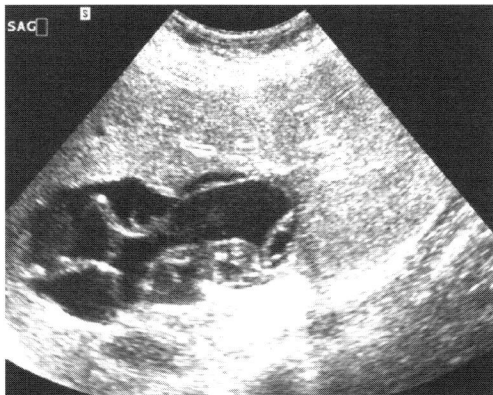

Figure 3. Ultrasound of the liver showing univesicular (Gharbi type 4) hydatid cyst with collapsed inner membrane.

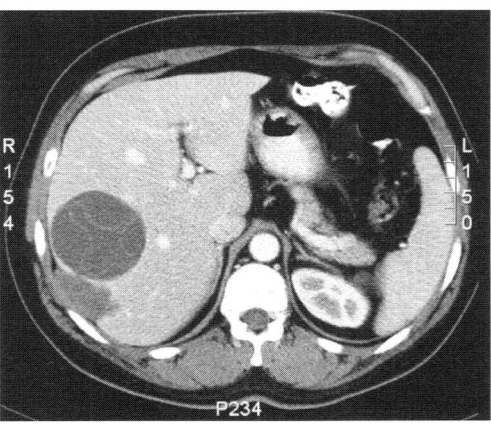

Figure 4. CT-scan of the liver showing univesicular hydatid cyst with collapsed inner membrane.

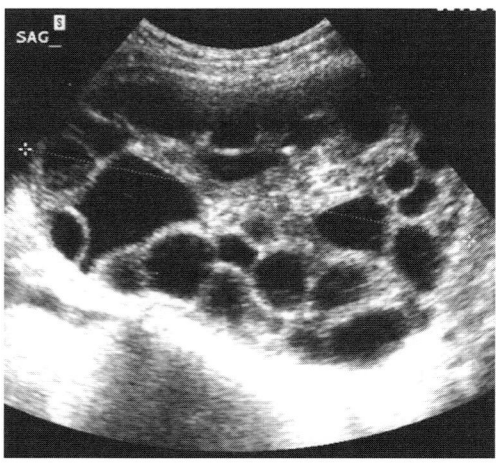

Figure 5. Ultrasound of the pelvic area showing a multivesicular hydatid cyst with multiple daughter cysts and amorphous material (so called "mother and daughter cyst").

Serology

ELISA is used as a screening test and IE (immuno-electrophoresis) as confirmation test. Diagnosis is established if both ELISA and IE are positive and likely if only ELISA is positive. Serology may be negative in 10-15% of cases, especially in well encapsulated cysts and pulmonary cysts.

Sensitivity for liver cysts is 80-90% and specificity 88-96%. Sensitivity is much lower when other organs are involved. For pulmonary cysts sensitivity is 50-56% and for other organ involvement 25-56%. IgG subclasses have been introduced to increase sensitivity. Specificity of IgG1 and IgG4 is high for echinococcosis and IgG4 response is more pronounced than that of IgG1. It has to be demonstrated yet that in cystic echinococcosis IgG4 is more sensitive for activity of the disease than IgG1 or total IgG [9-11].

Treatment

The ultimate goal of treatment is elimination of the germinal layer although the hydatid cyst itself and its mass effect on the surrounding liver tissue are the eye catchers. Currently, three treatment options are available (i) surgery, (ii) medical treatment and (iii) percutaneous treatment. Surgery was the only treatment option available until the mid 1980's. Then, medical treatment with mebendazole and albendazole was introduced. Since the early 1990's, a new percutaneous intervention is used for treatment of uncomplicated hydatid cysts with drainable content. This method was called PAIR, Puncture-Aspiration-Injection-Reaspiration. Later, PAIR-derived techniques were introduced for treatment of complicated hydatid cysts and cysts containing non-drainable material.

Surgery

The core principles of hydatid surgery are (i) total removal of all infective cyst parts and (ii) avoidance of intra-abdominal spillage of cyst content.

- **Radical surgical resection** (liver resection, pericystectomy and cystectomy) is the best prevention of intra-abdominal spillage. The hydatid cyst is entirely removed and opening of the hydatid cyst is avoided. Complication and recurrence rates are low. Liver resection, the most extensive technique, has comparable results to the less extensive methods of pericystectomy and cystectomy. Pericystectomy involves a non-anatomical resection of the entire hydatid cyst: the endocyst and the surrounding fibrous capsule (pericyst). This method is technically a more difficult procedure than cystectomy. In the view of experts, cystectomy is the procedure of choice. Cystectomy involves removal of the parasitic cyst or endocyst: laminar layer, germinal layer and cyst content. The pericyst (the fibrous capsule) is not resected [12-15].

- When radical surgery is impossible and surgical evacuation of cyst content is performed, intra-abdominal seeding of protoscoleces has to be avoided by additional measures. Peroperative use of scolecidals was introduced to lower the relapse rate. Hypertonic saline (15-30%), alcohol (70-95%), silver nitrate, cetrimide and others were used to irrigate the cyst cavity and the operation area. Saïdi introduced the "frozen seal", method in which cyst content and cyst wall are evacuated through a specially designed cone, frozen to the liver surface overlying the hydatid cyst. Walling of the operation field with gauzes soaked in hypertonic saline or other scolecidal agents is another less reliable method. Postoperative complication rates range from 8%-16%, relapse rate from 10%-30% and in-hospital mortality is 4%, depending on the method used [3, 16].

New development

Laparoscopic (peri) cystectomy or drainage of anteriorly located cysts was introduced as a new surgical technique. Compared to the classical approach by laparotomy, this method is less traumatic for the patient, requires a shorter hospital stay and recovery is faster. Results are encouraging even in complicated cases. During long-term follow-up, high success rates (77-100%) and low complication (0-17%) and recurrence rates (0-9%) were reported. However, this technique is limited to laparoscopically accessible cysts, mainly those located anteriorly in the liver. Expert consensus on indications and contraindications is needed [17-21].

Medical treatment

Benzimidazole carbamates (mebendazole and albendazole) are anthelmintic drugs that kill the parasite by impairing its glucose uptake. Benzimidazoles have proved effective against the larval stages of *Echinococcus granulosus*. From the early 1980s chemotherapy is used for treatment of human echinoccosis. Mebendazole was introduced first, but albendazole became the drug of choice due to its better absorption and better clinical results. Drugs were given in 3-month cycles interrupted after 28 days for two weeks. Medical treatment using interrupted cycles appeared to be parasitostatic rather than parasitocidal. Therefore, continuous daily treatment for a 3-month period was introduced [22].

Another basic problem was that most studies were not well designed, not prospective and not randomised. Therefore, treatment results of the older studies in the past 20 years are rather confusing. Success rates varied from 0-78% (median 30%) for mebendazole treated patients and from 30-88% (median 71%) for albendazole treated patients. At best, one-third of patients had been cured of their disease (complete and permanent disappearance of cysts) and 30-50% had responded with significant regression of cyst size and alleviation of symptoms [1, 23-26].

Recent well designed prospective randomised studies, demonstrated what may be expected from benzimidazole treatment. Patients with one single hydatid cyst were treated with mebendazole or albendazole for a period of three-six months. At 22 (12-170) months follow-up, success rate was 74% in all patients. The efficacy of albendazole (82%) was superior to that of mebendazole (56%). Relapse rate was 25% in both treatment groups. Most relapses (78%) occurred within two years after the end of treatment. More than 90% of these cysts responded well to additional courses of benzimidazoles. An important finding was that this study illustrated the necessity for extended post-treatment monitoring: 22% of relapses occurred between two and eight years following treatment. Interestingly, this study confirmed clinical observations from retrospective studies in the past that multivesicular cysts, hepatic cysts and cysts in older patients responded less well to treatment than univesicular cysts, pulmonary cysts respectively cysts in younger patients (< 30 years of age) [27-29].

The efficacy of preoperative albendazole treatment was established by two studies.

In a Chinese study, cyst viability after 3-month albendazole pre-treatment was 8% at the time of surgery, significantly lower than in the control group (100%). In a Spanish study, both a 1-month and a 3-month preoperative course of albendazole significantly reduced cyst viability to 28% respectively 6%. In placebo treated patients, 50% of cysts were viable at surgery. Although there are no published data on the efficacy of perioperative prophylaxis, it is generally advised [30, 31].

Reassuringly, albendazole treatment appeared anyhow to be better than no treatment. The natural course of pulmonary hydatid cysts was prospectively studied by comparing albendazole treatment with placebo. The efficacy of albendazole (71%) was superior to that of placebo (15.4%) [32].

Involution characteristics

Following benzimidazole treatment, most characteristic signs of involution are: (i) decrease of cyst size; (ii) detachment and collapse of inner membrane, sometimes showing a "water Lilly" sign; (iii) increase of echodensity and pseudosolidification of cyst content; (iv) cyst wall calcifications usually occur in a late stage.

Pharmacokinetics of albendazole

Treatment result may be improved when albendazole is properly dosed and administered. Pharmacokinetic studies demonstrated that albendazole absorption is variable from person to person and even within the same individual variability may be high. Gastric acidity and intestinal degradation are main factors determining albendazole absorption. Gastric pH is the first determinant of albendazole absorption. When administered on an empty stomach, absorption is highly variable from person to person, very probably due to the difference in gastric pH. Cimetidine decreases gastric acidity and thereby interindividual variability but also decreases albendazole absorption by 50%. The clinical observation that co-administration of albendazole with cimetidine improved treatment results cannot be understood from what we learned from pharmacokinetic studies.

Albendazole degradation in the lumen of the small intestine by cytochrome p-450 enzymes located in the villi is the second determinant of albendazole absorption. This process is variable from person to person because of the variable presence of these brush border enzymes. Intraluminal degradation can be inhibited by grapefruit juice constituents such as naringin and dihydroxybergamottin, resulting in a 3 fold increase of albendazole sulphoxide levels. After absorption, albendazole is rapidly metabolised by the liver into the active metabolite albendazole sulphoxide. This so-called "first pass" effect in the liver is approximately 100%. Albendazole absorption can be significantly improved by combining it with a fatty meal (4-9 fold) or with praziquantel (3 fold) or by administration of higher doses albendazole (10 mg/kg) [33-38].

For clinical practice, albendazole should better be administered in a higher dose (10 mg/kg, twice daily), combined with a meal (breakfast and diner) and better not be co-administered with drugs that reduce gastric acidity. Grapefruit juice may further support albendazole treatment. However, these practical advises are not yet supported by clinical studies demonstrating better outcome.

Adverse events of benzimidazole treatment were reported in 5.8-12.3% of patients treated. General complaints are headache, nausea, anorexia, vomiting, abdominal pain and itching. In the first weeks of treatment a transient increase of liver enzymes may be observed. Leucopenia is rare. In the course of treatment complete hair loss may occur, a very debilitating complication especially in women. Fortunately, hair growth reoccurs when albendazole is stopped. In 3-4% of patients albendazole had to be stopped due to intolerable adverse events. Albendazole should not be administered in the first trimester of pregnancy. Administration to pregnant sheep appeared to be teratogenic and embryotoxic.

New development

Recently, new albendazole formulations were used in a pharmacokinetic study in human volunteers. The relative bioavailability of albendazole formulations that use arachis oil-polysorbate 80 or hydroxypropyl-beta-cyclodextrin as an excipient was enhanced 4.3- and 9.7-fold compared to the results seen with commercial tablets [39].

In summary, medical treatment is focused on killing of the protoscoleces and on destruction of the germinal layer. The latter cannot be achieved in all cases. From what we know today, four different goals can be pursued with albendazole medication: definite cure, reduction of cyst viability, preoperative treatment and perioperative prophylaxis.

- **Definite cure of univesicular cysts**. Following a 3-6 month course, success rate is 82% and relapse rate 25%, most relapses occurring within 2 years after treatment. Life-long follow-up is advised for these patients.

- **Reduction of viability and of cyst size** is mostly the best what can be achieved in multivesicular cysts. The germinal layer is rather resistant to treatment. Peripheral daughter cysts remain viable or reappear from the germinal layer after treatment is stopped. The central part of the cyst becomes amorphous during treatment *(figure 6)*. Definite cure of multivesicular cysts occurs infrequently.

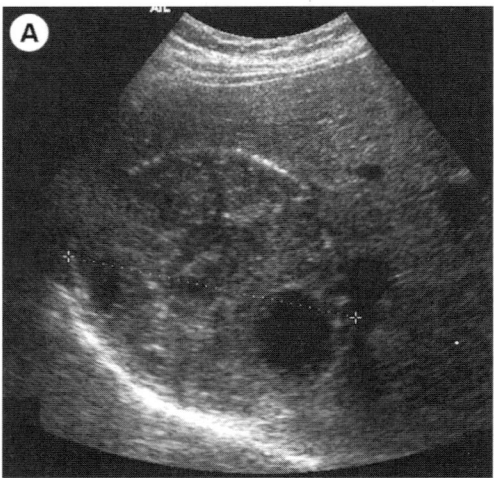
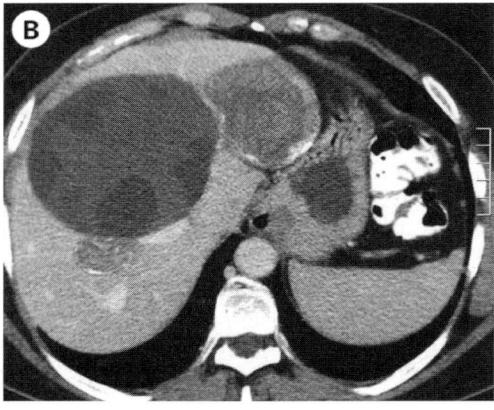

Figure 6. Ultrasound (A) and CT-scan (B) of a hepatic multivesicular hydatid cyst following multiple courses of albendazole. A typical pattern is shown: central amorphous mass, peripheral daughter cysts adjacent to the germinal layer and cyst wall calcifications.

- **Preoperative reduction of viability of univesicular cysts** when elective surgical or percutaneous treatment is planned.

- **Perioperative or peri-interventional prophylaxis**. Prophylaxis should optimally start at least three days before the surgical or percutaneous treatment. In urgent cases immediately before or after the intervention. Advises for post-treatment prophylaxis range from three-eight weeks for uncomplicated cases. In complicated cases with higher risk for spillage of cyst content three-six months are arbitrarily advised.

Percutaneous treatment

Percutaneous puncture of hydatid cysts has long been discouraged because of the risk of anaphylaxis and intraperitoneal seeding. Nevertheless, accidental and intended puncture of what appeared to be hydatid cysts happened to occur uneventful. The first successful report on percutaneous drainage of a hydatid cyst nicely illustrated the stepwise approach and the management of bile leakage. Fluoroscopy was used to puncture the cyst. A pigtail catheter was introduced to aspirate cyst fluid and inject silver nitrate and hypertonic saline.

Silver nitrate was regularly injected until aspirated protoscoleces had become non-viable. Cystography revealed a communication with the biliary tree. Patient was discharged with the drainage catheter in place. Weekly follow-up continued with concomitant silver nitrate irrigation of the cavity. After three months catheter was removed when daily bile drainage had decreased to < 5 ml [40].

In early 1990, a systematic percutaneous technique was introduced. To prevent intra-abdominal seeding, the hydatid cyst is punctured through normal liver tissue. The liver tissue collapses when needle or catheter is removed and thus serves as a protection against leakage of cyst fluid. This technique was based on that introduced for percutaneous treatment of non-parasitic cysts with 95% alcohol and called PAIR: Puncture-Aspiration-Injection-Reaspiration. Usually albendazole prophylaxis is started one week before PAIR and continued for three-four weeks thereafter. Briefly, in PAIR the cyst is punctured under US-guidance; cyst fluid is subtotally aspirated; 95% alcohol or hypertonic saline is injected; scolecidals are reaspirated after 10 minutes. Following intracystic injection of scolecidals both germinal layer and protoscoleces become instantaneously non-viable. Success of PAIR is defined as detachment of endocyst, rupture of daughter cysts and no viable protoscoleces at microscopy of cyst fluid. The most characteristic sonographic signs of involution at follow-up are: (i) heterogeneous reflections of cyst content (three months); (ii) obliteration and pseudotumor aspect (five months); (iii) loss of echogenicity and disappearance of cyst (nine months) [41, 42].

Many studies demonstrated that PAIR is safe, successful in 90-100% and has few relapses (0-4%) [43-47]. The WHO Informal Working Group on Echinococcosis reported the results of 765 hydatid cysts treated in multiple centres. In all but two cases at least 50% reduction in size and involution of the cysts were observed at long-term follow-up. Success rate was 99.7%, failure rate 0.26%, relapse rate 1.57% and complication rate 14.8%. Anaphylactic shock (one patient died) and spillage occurred in 0.52% each. Minor complications were observed in 13.7% [48].

Pioneers in the field of PAIR reported what may be expected from PAIR in experienced hands. At 59 (6-158) months follow-up of 52 patients with 65 hydatid cysts, success rate was 48% (> 50% reduction of cyst size; homogeneous solidification of content), partial success rate 35.4% (< 50% smaller; heterogeneous content), failure rate 16.6% (no morphologic changes; reappearance of daughter cysts) and complication rate was 13.8% (fever and urticaria only). No relapses occurred [49]. Others reported comparable results: success rate 93%, failure rate 7%, relapse rate 5%, complication rate 9%. One of the 78 treated patients died [50].

New developments

A simplified PAIR method using a mixture of alcohol 95% and polidocanol 1% (ethoxysclerol) proved to be safe and effective as well. Polidocanol was chosen as a sclerosing agent to destroy the germinal layer of the cyst and to enhance the sclerosing effect of alcohol. After ultrasound guided puncture, cyst fluid was drained freely until it ceased and simply replaced by a mixture of absolute alcohol and polidocanol. The needle was left five minutes inside the cyst and then withdrawn without reaspiration of scolecidals. Treatment was performed as an outpatient procedure without albendazole prophylaxis. Eighty-seven patients with 98 hydatid cysts (type 1, type 2 and type 3) were treated. At

33 months follow-up, cyst size significantly decreased from 7.7 cm to 6.3 cm. Moreover, 90% of cysts showed sonographically evidence of degeneration. The cavity was entirely filled with a solid echo pattern (33%) or partially filled with a pseudotumor pattern (58%) whereas no pseudotumor appearance was observed in 8% of treated cysts. Recurrence rate was 1% while no albendazole prophylaxis was used. One patient died due to an anaphylactic shock. The advantages of this procedure are: (i) it is simple and does not necessitate hospitalisation; (ii) unlike in PAIR, daughter cysts do not have to be punctured separately; (iii) albendazole prophylaxis is not necessary. The disadvantage is that reduction of mass effect, if necessary, is not very prominent [51].

However, PAIR and PAIR-like methods are contraindicated in patients with cystobiliary fistulas because scolecidals may cause sclerosing cholangitis [52-54]. For these complicated cases a new technique was developed: PEVAC, Percutaneous EVACuation of cyst content. Briefly, in PEVAC cyst is punctured under ultrasound guidance. Cyst fluid is aspirated to release intracystic pressure. A large bore catheter and sheath are inserted. Cyst content (daughter cysts, germinal layer and amorphous material) is evacuated by repeated injection and reaspiration of isotonic saline. Cystography checks for a possible cystobiliary (CB) fistula. CB-fistulas are treated by external drainage combined with endoprosthesis or sphincterotomy. Catheter is removed after complete cyst collapse and/or closure of the CB-fistula. Albendazole is started one week before PEVAC and continued for eight weeks thereafter. So far, a small number of patients have been treated with PEVAC but the results are encouraging. In all thirty patients, initial cyst size was 11.4 (6-21) cm. At 23 (3-50) months follow-up, twenty cysts had disappeared and ten cysts had decreased to 5.4 (2-9.4) cm, about 50% of the initial value. CB-fistulas (17 patients) and infections (22 patients) were the main complications. Allergic reactions (transient fever, skin rash and eosinophilia) were observed in three patients. Catheter-time and hospital stay was largely determined by the presence of a CB-fistula. Improvement on the management of CB-fistulas with earlier closure would significantly reduce patient morbidity. PEVAC is safe, effective and the intervention is not very complicated. PEVAC should better not be applied in cysts with massive extrahepatic extension [55].

A similar technique was reported to be effective in predominantly solid hydatid cyst, known to be most difficult to treat via the percutaneous route [56]. For treatment of multivesicular cysts, a cutting instrument was developed to facilitate the evacuation of daughter cysts and laminated membrane. In 90% of cases one single intervention was effective. Complication rate was 3%. At 9-48 months follow-up, no recurrences were observed in 32 treated patients [57, 58]. An impressive report from China in 1,409 patients with 1,614 cysts, confirmed the usefulness of percutaneous evacuation in general practice. The intervention failed in 1.86%, anaphylactic reactions were remarkably low (0.14%). Bile leakage occurred in 392 cysts (24%) necessitating a drainage time of 4-17 weeks. Surgery was necessary in 16 patients with bile leakage. At three years follow-up, relapse rate was 3.3% and success rate 98% [59].

Radiofrequency thermal ablation (RFTA) is an interesting experimental approach. This technique focuses on prevalently solid echinococcal cysts in the liver and is suggested to be an alternative treatment for PEVAC. So far, four patients have been treated with RFTA preceded by multiple courses of albendazole. The five cysts demonstrated a pattern typically seen following long-term albendazole treatment: solidification of the central part and small, peripheral daughter cysts *(figure 6)*. The RFTA needle electrodes were introduced under ultrasound guidance. Daughter cysts were broken by deploying the electrodes. Electrodes were placed adjacent to the germinal layer, the primary target of treatment. Energy was applied and temperature inside the cyst reached about $100°C$. After the procedure, cyst material was aspirated for microscopy. No protoscoleces or germinal layer could be identified. The results are preliminary and efficacy of RFTA has to be proven yet [60, 61].

Which treatment is the best?

Surgery, percutaneous treatment or medical treatment? An answer might be derived from studies directly comparing these treatment options and from a meta-analysis.

In one single centre, PAIR was compared with albendazole treatment and PAIR with surgery, in two different prospectively randomised studies. Multicenter studies on this topic are not available.

Albendazole monotherapy (ABZ; 10 mg/kg/d; 8 weeks) was compared with PAIR combined with albendazole (PAIR-ABZ) and with PAIR without it (PAIR). At six-nine months follow-up, results in the PAIR and PAIR-ABZ groups were superior to those in the ABZ group. In all PAIR and PAIR-ABZ treated patients complaints had disappeared and cysts had become significantly smaller, showing involution at ultrasonography. Remarkably, results in the PAIR-ABZ group were significantly better than those in the PAIR group. In the ABZ group, complaints had disappeared in a minority of patients, none of the cysts had become smaller and involution was present in a few cysts only. PAIR related complications were urticaria (2), transient fever (5), cyst infection (2) and cystobiliary fistula (1). It was concluded that (i) PAIR and PAIR-ABZ were superior to an eight weeks course of albendazole and (ii) PAIR-ABZ had significantly better results than PAIR [41].

PAIR and surgery were equally effective in reducing cyst size and causing disappearance of the cyst at 17 months follow-up. Following PAIR, mean cyst size decreased from 8.0 cm to 1.4 cm and following surgery from 9.1 cm to 0.9 cm. In the PAIR group 88% of cysts disappeared and in the surgery group 72%. The advantage of PAIR included a significantly shorter hospital stay (4.2 days *versus* 12.7 days) and a significantly lower complication rate (32% *versus* 84%). Recurrences and evidence of secondary growth of cysts were not observed [62].

In a recent meta-analysis, the clinical outcomes for 769 patients with hepatic cystic echinococcosis treated with percutaneous aspiration-injection-reaspiration (PAIR) plus albendazole or mebendazole was compared with 952 era-matched historical control subjects undergoing surgical intervention. The rate of clinical and parasitologic cure was greater in patients receiving PAIR plus chemotherapy (96% *vs* 90%). Disease recurrence (1.6% *vs* 6.3%), major complications (8% *vs* 25%), minor complications (13% *vs* 33%) and death (0.1% *vs* 0.7%) occurred more frequently among surgical control subjects. Fever and minor allergic reactions subjects were more common among PAIR-treated subjects. The mean durations of hospital stay were 2.4 days for the PAIR-group and 15.0 days for the surgery-group. Compared with surgery, PAIR plus chemotherapy is associated with greater clinical and parasitologic efficacy; lower rates of morbidity, mortality, and disease recurrence; and shorter hospital stays [63].

Conclusion

Modern management of echinoccosis needs the availability of all three treatment options: medical treatment, percutaneous treatment and surgery. Surgery is no longer the treatment of first choice for hepatic echinococcosis. In patients with univesicular cysts, albendazole monotherapy is the first choice. PAIR is indicated when pain is intractable or albendazole fails. In patients with multivesicular cysts, PEVAC is a better choice. Percutaneous treatment with a combination of alcohol and polidocanol may be used instead of PAIR or PEVAC, but not in cases associated with cystobiliary fistulas. Surgery is the first choice only when: (i) expertise of percutaneous treatment is not available; (ii) percutaneous treatment cannot be safely undertaken; and (iii) significant extrahepatic extension of the cyst is associated with a high risk of perforation or precludes adequate percutaneous treatment; (iv) in case of a rupture into the peritoneal cavity.

Take home messages

- Geography, imaging and serology are the keystones of the diagnosis echinococcosis.

- Medical treatment takes months, follow-up years and relapse rate is high.

- Percutaneous treatment replaces surgery in cases with limited extrahepatic extension.

References

1. Schipper HG, Kager PA. Diagnosis and treatment of unilocular hydatid disease (Echinococcus granulosus infection). *Ned Tijdschr Geneeskd* 1997; 141: 984-9.
2. Wen H, New RR, Craig PS. Diagnosis and treatment of human hydatidosis. *Br J Clin Pharmacol* 1993; 35: 565-74.
3. Kammerer WS, Schantz PM. Echinococcal disease. *Infect Dis Clin North Am* 1993; 7: 605-18.
4. Yahya AI, Przybylski J, Foud A. Anaphylactic shock in a patient with ruptured hydatid liver cyst owing to trivial abdominal trauma. *J R Coll Surg Edinb* 1997; 42: 423-4.
5. Horzic M, Bunoza D, Maric K. Anaphylactic shock in a female patient due to a spontaneous rupture of a hepatic hydatid cyst: a case report. *Hepatogastroenterology* 1996; 43: 1601-2.
6. Mooraki A, Rahbar MH, Bastani B. Spontaneous systemic anaphylaxis as an unusual presentation of hydatid cyst: report of two cases. *Am J Trop Med Hyg* 1996; 55: 302-3.
7. Kok AN, Yurtman T, Aydin NE. Sudden death due to ruptured hydatid cyst of the liver. *J Forensic Sci* 1993; 38: 978-80.
8. Gharbi HA, Hassine W, Brauner MW, Dupuch K. Ultrasound examination of the hydatic liver. *Radiology* 1981; 139: 459-63.

9. Shambesh MK, Craig PS, Wen H, Rogan MT, Paolillo E. IgG1 and IgG4 serum antibody responses in asymptomatic and clinically expressed cystic echinococcosis patients. *Acta Trop* 1997; 64: 53-63.
10. Wen H, Bresson-Hadni S, Vuitton DA, Lenys D, Yang BM, Ding ZX, et al. Analysis of immunoglobulin G subclass in the serum antibody responses of alveolar echinococcosis patients after surgical treatment and chemotherapy as an aid to assessing the outcome. *Trans R Soc Trop Med Hyg* 1995; 89: 692-7.
11. Wen H, Craig PS. Immunoglobulin G subclass responses in human cystic and alveolar echinococcosis. *Am J Trop Med Hyg* 1994; 51: 741-8.
12. Alfieri S, Doglietto GB, Pacelli F, Costamagna G, Carriero C, Mutignani M, et al. Radical surgery for liver hydatid disease: a study of 89 consecutive patients. *Hepatogastroenterology* 1997; 44: 496-500.
13. Ammori BJ, Jenkins BL, Lim PC, Prasad KR, Pollard SG, Lodge JP. Surgical strategy for cystic diseases of the liver in a western hepatobiliary center. *World J Surg* 2002; 26: 462-9.
14. Fenton-Lee D, Morris DL. The management of hydatid disease of the liver: Part 2. *Trop Doct* 1997; 27: 87-8.
15. Fenton-Lee D, Morris DL. The management of hydatid disease of the liver: Part 1. *Trop Doct* 1996; 26: 173-6.
16. Saidi F. A new approach to the surgical treatment of hydatid cyst. *Ann R Coll Surg Engl* 1977; 59: 115-8.
17. Bickel A, Loberant N, Singer-Jordan J, Goldfeld M, Daud G, Eitan A. The laparoscopic approach to abdominal hydatid cysts: a prospective nonselective study using the isolated hypobaric technique. *Arch Surg* 2001; 136: 789-95.
18. Khoury G, Abiad F, Geagea T, Nabout G, Jabbour S. Laparoscopic treatment of hydatid cysts of the liver and spleen. *Surg Endosc* 2000; 14: 243-5.
19. Manterola C, Fernandez O, Munoz S, Vial M, Losada H, Carrasco R, et al. Laparoscopic pericystectomy for liver hydatid cysts. *Surg Endosc* 2002; 16: 521-4.
20. Seven R, Berber E, Mercan S, Eminoglu L, Budak D. Laparoscopic treatment of hepatic hydatid cysts. *Surgery* 2000; 128: 36-40.
21. Sgourakis G, Gemos K, Dedemadi G, Spetzouris N, Gyftakis H, Salapa P. Laparoscopic drainage of infected hydatid liver cysts. *Minerva Chir* 2001; 56: 169-73.
22. Schantz PM, Van den Bossche H, Eckert J. Chemotherapy for larval echinococcosis in animals and humans: report of a workshop. *Z Parasitenkd* 1982; 67: 5-26.
23. Horton RJ. Albendazole in treatment of human cystic echinococcosis: 12 years of experience. *Acta Trop* 1997; 64: 79-93.
24. Teggi A, Lastilla MG, De Rosa F. Therapy of human hydatid disease with mebendazole and albendazole. *Antimicrob Agents Chemother* 1993; 37: 1679-84.
25. Todorov T, Vutova K, Mechkov G, Petkov D, Nedelkov G, Tonchev Z. Evaluation of response to chemotherapy of human cystic echinococcosis. *Br J Radiol* 1990; 63: 523-31.
26. Davis A, Dixon H, Pawlowski ZS. Multicentre clinical trials of benzimidazole-carbamates in human cystic echinococcosis (phase 2). *Bull World Health Organ* 1989; 67: 503-8.
27. Franchi C, Di Vico B, Teggi A. Long-term evaluation of patients with hydatidosis treated with benzimidazole carbamates. *Clin Infect Dis* 1999; 29: 304-9.
28. Todorov T, Mechkov G, Vutova K, Georgiev P, Lazarova I, Tonchev Z, et al. Factors influencing the response to chemotherapy in human cystic echinococcosis. *Bull World Health Organ* 1992; 70: 347-58.
29. Schantz PM. Editorial response: Treatment of cystic echinococcosis – improving but still limited. *Clin Infect Dis* 1999; 29: 310-1.
30. Gil-Grande LA, Rodriguez-Caabeiro F, Prieto JG, Sanchez-Ruano JJ, Brasa C, Aguilar L, et al. Randomised controlled trial of efficacy of albendazole in intra-abdominal hydatid disease. *Lancet* 1993; 342: 1269-72.

31. Wen H, Zou PF, Yang WG, Lu J, Wang YH, Zhang JH, *et al.* Albendazole chemotherapy for human cystic and alveolar echinococcosis in north-western China. *Trans R Soc Trop Med Hyg* 1994; 88: 340-3.
32. Keshmiri M, Baharvahdat H, Fattahi SH, Davachi B, Dabiri RH, Baradaran H, *et al.* A placebo controlled study of albendazole in the treatment of pulmonary echinococcosis. *Eur Respir J* 1999; 14: 503-7.
33. Awadzi K, Hero M, Opoku NO, Buttner DW, Coventry PA, Prime MA, *et al.* The chemotherapy of onchocerciasis XVII. A clinical evaluation of albendazole in patients with onchocerciasis; effects of food and pretreatment with ivermectin on drug response and pharmacokinetics. *Trop Med Parasitol* 1994; 45: 203-8.
34. Lange H, Eggers R, Bircher J. Increased systemic availability of albendazole when taken with a fatty meal. *Eur J Clin Pharmacol* 1988; 34: 315-7.
35. Gottschall dw, Theodorides VJ, Wang R. The metabolism of benzimidazole anthelmintics. *Parasitology Today* 1999 : 115-24.
36. Nagy J, Schipper HG, Koopmans RP, Butter JJ, Van Boxtel CJ, Kager PA. Effect of grapefruit juice or cimetidine coadministration on albendazole bioavailability. *Am J Trop Med Hyg* 2002; 66: 260-3.
37. Schipper HG, Koopmans RP, Nagy J, Butter JJ, Kager PA, Van Boxtel CJ. Effect of dose increase or cimetidine co-administration on albendazole bioavailability. *Am J Trop Med Hyg* 2000; 63: 270-3.
38. Wen H, Zhang HW, Muhmut M, Zou PF, New RR, Craig PS. Initial observation on albendazole in combination with cimetidine for the treatment of human cystic echinococcosis. *Ann Trop Med Parasitol* 1994; 88: 49-52.
39. Rigter IM, Schipper HG, Koopmans RP, van Kan HJ, Frijlink HW, Kager PA, *et al.* Relative bioavailability of three newly developed albendazole formulations: a randomized crossover study with healthy volunteers. *Antimicrob Agents Chemother* 2004; 48: 1051-4.
40. Mueller PR, Dawson SL, Ferrucci JT, Jr., Nardi GL. Hepatic echinococcal cyst: successful percutaneous drainage. *Radiology* 1985; 155: 627-8.
41. Khuroo MS, Dar MY, Yattoo GN, Zargar SA, Javaid G, Khan BA, *et al.* Percutaneous drainage *versus* albendazole therapy in hepatic hydatidosis: a prospective, randomized study. *Gastroenterology* 1993; 104: 1452-9.
42. Bret PM, Fond A, Bretagnolle M, Valette PJ, Thiesse P, Lambert R, *et al.* Percutaneous aspiration and drainage of hydatid cysts in the liver. *Radiology* 1988; 168: 617-20.
43. Akhan O, Ozmen MN. Percutaneous treatment of liver hydatid cysts. [Review] [55 refs]. *Eur J Radiol* 1999; 32: 76-85.
44. Filice C, Pirola F, Brunetti E, Dughetti S, Strosselli M, Foglieni, *et al.* A new therapeutic approach for hydatid liver cysts. Aspiration and alcohol injection under sonographic guidance. *Gastroenterology* 1990; 98: 1366-8.
45. Giorgio A, Tarantino L, Francica G, Mariniello N, Aloisio T, Soscia, *et al.* Unilocular hydatid liver cysts: treatment with US-guided, double percutaneous aspiration and alcohol injection. *Radiology* 1992; 184: 705-10.
46. Khuroo MS, Zargar SA, Mahajan R. Echinococcus granulosus cysts in the liver: management with percutaneous drainage. *Radiology* 1991; 180: 141-5.
47. Salama H, Farid A, Strickland GT. Diagnosis and treatment of hepatic hydatid cysts with the aid of echo-guided percutaneous cyst puncture. *Clin Infect Dis* 1995; 21: 1372-6.
48. Filice C, Brunetti E, Bruno R, Crippa FG, WHO-Informal Working Group on Echinococcosis-PAIR Network. Percutaneous drainage of echinococcal cysts (PAIR-puncture, aspiration, injection, reaspiration): results of a worldwide survey for assessment of its safety and efficacy. *Gut* 2000; 47: 156-7.
49. Garlaschelli A, Marangio A, Gulizia R, Filice C, Brunetti E. PAIR for abdominal cystic echinococcosis: results of a 15 year experience as a contribution to an evidence-based management of the disease. *Acta Tropica* 2002 : S91-2.

50. Giorgio A, Tarantino L, de Stefano G, Francica G, Mariniello N, Farella N, *et al.* Hydatid liver cyst: an 11-year experience of treatment with percutaneous aspiration and ethanol injection. *J Ultrasound Med* 2001; 20: 729-38.
51. Ormeci N, Soykan I, Bektas A, Sanoglu M, Palabiyikoglu M, Hadi YM, *et al.* A new percutaneous approach for the treatment of hydatid cysts of the liver. *Am J Gastroenterol* 2001; 96: 2225-30.
52. Castellano G, Moreno-Sanchez D, Gutierrez J, Moreno-Gonzalez E, Colina, Solis-Herruzo JA. Caustic sclerosing cholangitis. Report of four cases and a cumulative review of the literature. *Hepatogastroenterology* 1994; 41: 458-70.
53. Belghiti J, Benhamou JP, Houry S, Grenier P, Huguier M, Fekete F. Caustic sclerosing cholangitis. A complication of the surgical treatment of hydatid disease of the liver. *Arch Surg* 1986; 121: 1162-5.
54. Teres J, Gomez-Moli J, Bruguera M, Visa J, Bordas JM, Pera C. Sclerosing cholangitis after surgical treatment of hepatic echinococcal cysts. Report of three cases. *Am J Surg* 1984; 148: 694-7.
55. Schipper HG, Lameris JS, van Delden OM, Rauws EA, Kager PA. Percutaneous evacuation (PEVAC) of multivesicular echinococcal cysts with or without cystobiliary fistulas which contain non-drainable material: first results of a modified PAIR method. *Gut* 2002; 50: 718-23.
56. Haddad MC, Sammak BM, Al Karawi M. Percutaneous treatment of heterogenous predominantly solid echopattern echinococcal cysts of the liver. *Cardiovasc Intervent Radiol* 2000; 23: 121-5.
57. Saremi F, McNamara TO. Hydatid cysts of the liver: long-term results of percutaneous treatment using a cutting instrument. *AJR Am J Roentgenol* 1995; 165: 1163-7.
58. Saremi F. Percutaneous drainage of hydatid cysts: use of a new cutting device to avoid leakage. *Am J Roentgenol* 1992; 158: 83-5.
59. Vuitton DA, Xiao Zhi Wang, Sheng Li Feng, Jing Sheng Chen, Yong Shou Li, Shu Fang Li, Qiong Ke Tang. PAIR-derived US-guided techniques for the treatment of cystic echinococcosis: a Chinese experience. *Gut e-Letter*, 18-7-2002.
60. Brunetti E, Filice C. Radiofrequency thermal ablation of echinococcal liver cysts. *Lancet* 2001; 358: 1464.
61. Brunetti E, Marangio A, Gulizia R, Filice C. Ultrasound-guided radiofrequency thermal ablation of prevalently solid echinococcal liver cysts. *Acta Tropica* 2002 : S90-1.
62. Khuroo MS, Wani NA, Javid G, Khan BA, Yattoo GN, Shah AH, *et al.* Percutaneous drainage compared with surgery for hepatic hydatid cysts. *N Engl J Med* 1997; 337: 881-7.
63. Smego RA, Bhatti S, Khaliq AA, Beg MA. Percutaneous aspiration-injection-reaspiration drainage plus albendazole or mebendazole for hepatic cystic echinococcosis: a meta-analysis. *Clin Infect Dis* 2003; 37: 1073-83.

Postoperative abscesses

Peter B. Soeters, W. van Gemert, C.H. Dejong, J.W. Greve

Department of Surgery, University of Maastricht, The Netherlands

Postoperative infection is a dreaded complication of abdominal surgery, leading to substantial morbidity and mortality. Knowledge of the risk factors, involved in the occurrence of postoperative infection should guide preoperative management and preparation for surgery, as well as the surgical approach itself, to minimize postoperative infection. Once abdominal infection has developed, its early recognition is essential to institute early therapy. Modern imaging techniques do not only allow delineation of the topography of the abscess(es) but also their drainage *via* minimally invasive techniques. Therapy for intraabdominal abscesses should be tailored to the individual health state of the patient and the local intraabdominal infection to acquire an optimal outcome and to limit morbidity and mortality. These issues will be discussed in this chapter.

Risk factors for abdominal septic complications

Bloodloss

Bloodloss and subsequent blood transfusion are by far the most important risk factors for the development of postoperative infectious complications and their severity [1, 2]. It is very likely that this is caused by the immunosuppressive effect of the blood components transfused and not to the extent of the surgical trauma [3]. It is of interest that a storage time of the blood transfused, longer than 21 days, was associated with an increased risk to develop postoperative septic complications [4].

Weight loss

In 1936 Studley was the first to report an increased mortality in patients operated for peptic ulcer disease, who had lost 10-15% of their body weight before operation [5]. This has been found repeatedly thereafter. Importantly the severity of infectious complications can be limited by a preoperative 7-10-day course of nutritional rehabilitation in patients that have lost more than 10% of their body weight in the six months before operation, and who are not suffering from active infection [6].

Organ failure

Survival from septic postoperative complications is dependent on the health state of the patient before operation. The health state is not only determined by nutritional state (*see* "Weight loss") but also by organ function, or the lack thereof. To adequately respond to the septic state the patient needs to be able to generate a hyperdynamic circulation in the presence of increased metabolic demands, which requires good cardio-respiratory function. If the patient is suffering from heart or lung disease and cannot increase cardiac output and oxygen uptake, outcome is negatively affected [7].

The liver is crucially involved in the response to trauma and infection. It harbours a great number of Kupffer cells, and synthesises many acute phase proteins (opsonins, complement factors, clotting factors, albumin, fibrinogen, globulins). It has been demonstrated that septic liver patients die, when they are not able to take up sufficient quantities of amino acids to synthesise all these components [8, 9]. In a recent survey it was found that in patients with liver disease the complication rate after cholecystectomy was significantly raised [10]. The increased morbidity most likely should be explained by the fact that patients with liver insufficiency bleed more easily and respond less well to surgical trauma. A contributing factor to the increase in morbidity consists of the fact that cholecystectomy in liver patients is more often performed for acute cholecystitis [10].

Intoxications/drugs

Smoking and alcohol abuse have been found to be associated with increased infectious morbidity and mortality [11, 12]. The underlying mechanisms are unclear, although restrictive lung disease induced by smoking and diminished liver function induced by alcohol abuse are likely causes. Smoking does also appear to have a more generalized deleterious effect on host response, because it does not only increase the likelihood of developing pulmonary infectious complications after operation, but also infectious complications in the operative field [11].

Immunomodulatory drugs have been claimed to decrease healing rates after operations. This was not confirmed in patients with Crohn's disease [13]. Steroids may especially increase the severity of infectious complications, because the steroid delays adequate walling off of leaking anastomoses and abscesses. In addition clinical signs of infectious complications are often mitigated, which delays rapid diagnosis and therapy.

Inflammation/Infection

A strong correlation has been found between the degree of contamination, ranging from clean to generalized peritonitis, and the risk of post-operative intra-abdominal infection and mortality [14-16]. Hinchey has proposed a categorisation which also takes into account more general symptoms of infection [17, 18]. In patients that have clear signs of infection before operation (Hinchey stage III, IV) postoperative infection rates rise precipitously [17].

These findings are supported by earlier findings in the past decades, showing strong correlations between the acute phase response and postoperative complications. At present consensus is growing that plasma albumin levels do decrease as a result of the stress response rather than of nutritional depletion. Consequently the inflammatory state should caution to adopt a defensive approach to surgery, because of the increased risk to develop septic complications [19].

Type of surgery

In the foregoing part of this manuscript risk factors have been described that increase the likelihood of developing septic complications. Taken together they imply that the extent of the surgical trauma should not exceed the capacity of the patient to raise an adequate host response to the trauma. This implies that the smaller the ability to raise an adequate host response, the smaller the surgical trauma should be.

Kirkpatrick suggests that primary repair of intra-operative bowel lesions achieves better healing than complete anastomosis [20]. Seprafilm has been demonstrated to prevent adhesions, but the data suggest also that it increases the anastomotic leakage rate [21]. Indeed healthy anastomotic healing requires a healthy surrounding matrix, and the increased leakage rate in patients treated with Seprafilm suggests that the preventive action on the formation of adhesions simultaneously inhibits healthy fibrinous healing of anastomoses [21]. There are a few recent reports on the potential increase in the occurrence of postoperative abscesses after laparoscopic appendectomy in children [22, 23]. However, another report does not show differences [24]. Although the data are not unequivocal, some caution appears to be warranted in the laparoscopic approach to appendectomy in children.

Preventive measures

Antibiotics

Several studies have implicated that the incidence of postoperative infections can be diminished by the perioperative administration of antibiotics. Whereas the choice of antibiotics in orthopaedic surgery should predominantly focus on skin flora, in abdominal surgery the choice should focus on the faecal flora. In a recent Cochrane report it was concluded that postoperative infection after appendectomy was diminished by pre-, peri- or postoperative administration of antibiotics [25]. Similary efficacy of antibiotic prophylaxis has been demonstrated for other types of abdominal surgery.

Treatment of local and generalized infection

Infection at the site of the future operation inhibits healthy healing of anastomoses and wounds. This is a generally felt and accepted finding in surgery. The evidence for it may be derived from the epidemiological finding that the MPI (Mannheim Peritonitis Index: *see earlier*) correlates with postoperative septic morbidity [16]. It is therefore of paramount importance that local infection is treated before operation if possible. Abscesses should be drained and parenchymatous infection should be treated with appropriate antibiotics. Adequate treatment of infection before operation allows the organism to become anabolic and to respond adequately to the renewed challenge of the operation. Signs of recovery from infection consist of loss of extracellular oedema (negative fluid balance), spontaneous rises of plasma albumin and hemoglobin and an improved sense of well being. Although in this phase body weight decreases due to the loss of edema, muscle protein and strength increase. These statements do apply even more during generalized infection (sepsis). Primary anastomoses should not be performed in the septic state, surgery should only be undertaken when there is no other possibility but the surgical approach should be as simple and defensive as possible. This often includes resection of the diseased area, and the construction of stomas rather than primary anastomoses.

Nutritional state

The severely depleted organism cannot raise a normal healing response. There is no normal fibrin formation at the site of anastomoses and wounds. Also the response to infection is abnormal in the sense that often no fever can be generated, no leucocytosis, no walling of infectious processes. This mitigated response to infection is even more dangerous because it delays diagnosis and consequently treatment of complications. Seven to ten-day courses of nutritional repletion appear to be sufficient to improve host response despite the fact that often muscle mass has not yet recovered [26]. Many nutritional regimens have been advocated to improve outcome from surgery. Apart from the benefit of preoperative nutrition in depleted patients immunonutrition appears to be useful in surgical patients. There are multimodality formulae containing RNA, arginine and omega 3-fatty acids, and formulae that contain extra glutamine. Especially septic morbidity appears to improve due to this type of intervention [27, 28]. Recently a Swedish group has advocated the use of preoperative glucose to diminish glucose intolerance and to reduce metabolic stress. It has been suggested that length of stay in the hospital will be reduced by this measure.

Bowel cleansing

Bowel cleansing has been strongly advocated in the past. Its efficacy appeared to have been proven, but the benefit most likely should be explained by the simultaneous use of prophylactic antibiotics. In prospective randomised studies no benefit was demonstrated in patients undergoing colo-rectal surgery [29, 30].

Surgical approach

It is generally accepted that surgical technique should be impeccable, including limitation of blood loss, working along anatomic planes if possible, and limitation of tissue damage and devascularisation. The experience with Seprafilm [21] supports the intuitive feeling of surgeons that anastomoses will only heal when they are surrounded by healthy tissue. A matrix is needed walling of the anastomosis and allowing a healthy fibrinous exudate to develop which serves as the basis for healthy anastomotic wound healing. To ensure that this happens, anastomoses or sutured defects in the bowel should not be exposed to denuded areas, foreign material (meshes, Seprafilm), or other anastomoses. Care should be taken that anastomoses are not exposed in open wounds in case of the likelihood of the development of abdominal wall dehiscences. Similarly neighbouring hematomas, pus collections, urinary or other leakage should be prevented or when there is a serious risk that they may develop, the anastomosis should be positioned in such a way that close contact is unlikely.

Some authors have furnished evidence that delayed wound closure may limit the risk and morbidity of wound infection [31], but others have not found a benefit of this approach.

Time course of septic complications after operation

For a correct diagnosis and rapid and adequate treatment of postoperative infection it is important to estimate the likelihood of which problems can be encountered at which stage after operation [32].

0-2 days after operation

After abdominal surgery an inflammatory response occurs. This includes a temperature rise, tachycardia, increased cardiac output, hyperventilation, a fluid shift leading to an increased extravascular extracellular volume, and abdominal pain. This stress response is however mitigated with optimal surgery and anaesthesia. These signs may also be caused by infection and the distinction between a normal postoperative response and infection may be difficult early after surgery. However, abdominal sepsis is very unlikely at this stage, but if present often represents a technical mistake. An example is small bowel leakage due to inadvertent laceration of the bowel, which is a more dramatic event than large bowel leakage. This may be due to the flui[PB1]dity of the bowel contents spilling into the abdominal cavity, which may rapidly give rise to generalised peritonitis and requires immediate relaparotomy. Atelectasis due to bowel distension and pain is much more likely to happen within 48 hours after operation and to cause an inflammatory responce. An important measure to prevent this consists of adequate pain treatment. Epidural analgesia does not require systemic opiates and therefore keeps patients alert and does not depress respiratory drive.

2-3 days after operation

At this stage of the operation the balance point should be reached. This implies that the retention of water and salt by the kidney and the sequestration of fluid in the extravascular and extracellular compartment reverse to a decrease of the volume of these compartments. This fluid shifts to the intravascular compartment and leads to an increase of the circulating intravascular volume, in turn leading to increased urine production. Patients with cardiac pump failure or chronic renal failure may develop lung oedema and dyspnoea, requiring diuretics and fluid restriction. At this stage after operation fever generally indicates atelectasis or pneumonia, but an intra-abdominal complication, such as an anastomotic leak, should be considered, particularly when the fluid balance is strongly positive, bowel movements have not been resumed and the patient does not recover. The earlier leakage occurs, the more serious it is and the more likely it is that it results from technical failure. At this stage infection may rapidly spread to the whole abdomen and cause a generalised peritonitis. In old or severely depleted patients and in patients receiving immunosuppressive medication clinical signs may be mitigated. Hypothermia is an ominous sign of sepsis and has a worse prognosis than patients that generate fever in response to their septic state [33].

3-6 days after operation

In this period the majority of infectious problems in the abdomen becomes overt. Bowel movements do not resume, the abdomen remains distended and painful. Paradoxical diarrhoea may occur, which is often interpreted as a sign of recovery and delays prompt diagnosis of abdominal sepsis. Sometimes pelvic pain and dysuria in concert with a positive urine culture, caused by an inflammatory mass in the pelvis secondary to anastomotic leakage is erroneously attributed to a urinary infection. Sudden diffuse abdominal pain after initial postoperative recovery indicates a walled off anastomotic leak which after a few days has perforated into the peritoneal cavity.

7-14 days after operation

In this period intra-abdominal abscesses are the main cause of abdominal sepsis. The infectious process is localized due to adherence of parts of the intestine. The symptomatology varies between spiking temperature and septic symptoms to slight fever and malaise, mild abdominal discomfort and normal vital signs.

Diagnosis of postoperative infection

Clinical diagnosis of infection

In the preceding section the time-related gravity and character of postoperative infection has been described. This should be born in mind when considering the cause of postoperative complications and its treatment. Wounds draining sero-sanguinous fluid or overt pus, wound dehiscence, presence of adynamic ileus, pain, malaise, and cardio-respiratory complications in the first week, no stool passage or paradoxical diarrhoea, fever and leucocytosis should all raise the suspicion of anastomotic leak [32]. Patients are ill, and not alert. The balance point is not reached, implying that they continue to be in a positive fluid balance, due to parenteral fluid administration, required to sustain blood pressure and urine production.

Imaging

Clinical suspicion of early postoperative infection should in general lead to immediate re-intervention, because the cause then is generally due to technical failure and the infection very likely will spread to the whole abdominal cavity. Statistically the likelihood of intra-abdominal infection within a few days after operation is low however, and the cause of inflammatory activity most often resides in the lungs as a result of pain, bad coughing and atelectasis. Chest X-rays therefore will generally show abnormalities in the lower lung fields. Ct-scanning and ultrasound are not very helpful in this stage in detecting infectious complications in the abdomen.

In the second half of the first week after operation intra-abdominal infection generally has become clinically manifest although this sometimes is only diagnosed in retrospect. Severe sepsis should still lead to re-intervention, but lower grade infectious symptoms may warrant a primary diagnostic approach. Ct-scanning with intravenous and enteral (oral and/or rectal) contrast enhancement are necessary to derive the full benefit of the scan. In upper GI surgery involving the (sub-)hepatic area ultrasound imaging may be diagnostic.

Seven to 14 days after operation intra-abdominal abscesses are the main cause of abdominal sepsis. Ct-scanning with enteral and parenteral contrast enhancement has been proven to have a higher diagnostic yield than scintigraphy with labelled leukocytes [34-36]. In the aged population Gallium scan has a higher diagnostic accuracy after colo-rectal surgery than CRP, WBC and fever, but clinical symptomatology is very likely superior as the basis for further diagnostic work-up [37].

When fluid collections are diagnosed by imaging techniques, contrast enhancement of the walls of the contrast provide strong evidence that the collection is an abscess. In newly developing abscesses but also in severely depleted patients contrast enhancement as a sign of an inflammatory response of the organs, walling of the abscess may be absent. Therefore sampling of the collection should be performed by ultrasound- or CT-guided puncture. Relatively simple clinical chemistry and microbiology investigations in the material obtained by puncture can help to establish the diagnosis *(table I)*. Small bowel contents always contain bilirubin, amylase, electrolytes and very low amounts of albumin. Bile does however not contain amylase, whereas pure pancreatic juice does not contain bilirubin. Ascites or serous collections contain substantial concentrations of albumin depending on the plasma level and on whether the ascites is infected. In some cases measurement of triglycerides, lymphocytes (chylus) or creatinine, urea (in urine) may establish the diagnosis. In colonic diarrhoea electrolytes may help to distinguish between secretory (high sodium) and osmotic (much lower sodium) diarrhoea. The use of acute Gram stains in the material obtained has been questioned. They may however provide evidence for infection in young abscesses or in patients that are not able to generate an active inflammatory response, especially when combined with clinical symptomatology [38]. Also microbiologic culture may yield micro-organisms in collections that appear to be sterile at first ultrasound or CT sight, and may predict the likelihood of abscess formation when *Streptococcus milleri* is found [39].

Table I. The origin of abdominal secretions as derived from their relative composition: Bilirubin (Bil), Pancrease, Albumin (Alb), Triglycerides (Triglyc)

Bile	Bil H	Pancrease L	Alb L	Triglyc L
Pancreatic juice	Bil L	Pancrease H	Alb L	Triglyc L
Small bowel content	Bil H	Pancrease H	Alb L	Triglyc L or H
Ascites	Bil L	Pancrease L	Alb H	Triglyc L
Chyle	Bil L	Pancrease L	Alb H	Triglyc H

H = high concentration; L = low concentration.

Therapy

Time course

The earlier the diagnosis is made, the earlier intervention is done, minimising the morbidity and mortality of this surgical complication. Simultaneously, the earlier severe septic symptoms occur, the more severe the intra-abdominal problem is, and the more promptly surgical intervention should be undertaken. The type of surgery at re-laparotomy depends on the severity of the local septic process, and on the condition of the patient. In patients with little metabolic reserve, including those with nutritional depletion or using steroids, the first objective is to allow the patient to survive. Therefore the least risky operation should be performed. This generally includes a breakdown of the leaking anastomosis and creation of an enterostomy or exteriorization of leaking bowel segments. However, the attending surgeon should take into consideration that a Hartman procedure after a high anterior resection is safe and also leaves open the possibility to restore continuity. This is not so easy in patients that have undergone low anterior resection with mesorectal excision and low anastomoses. Under those circumstances local drainage should be preferred when the septic process is localised and the patient is young and at low risk [40]. The leaking bowel may be drained, closed or resected with primary re-anastomosis or suturing of the defect, preferably protected by a proximal diverting enterostomy [41].

After one week intra-abdominal abscesses are the main cause of abdominal sepsis.

The infectious process is localized due to adherence of parts of the intestine. The symptomatology varies between spiking temperature and septic symptoms to slight fever and malaise, mild abdominal discomfort and normal vital signs. In patients with mild symptoms a conservative approach, including appropriate antibiotics, may be warranted. A more aggressive policy is needed in case of septic signs.

Small anastomotic failure with an adjacent unilocular abscess of greater size (approximately 5 cm in diameter or larger) generally needs drainage either internally *via* the anastomosis, or externally *via* CT scan or US guided puncture and drainage. Such leakage sometimes requires a diverting loop ileostomy or colostomy. However, the decision to perform a relaparotomy should not be taken liberally, since secondary morbidity is extensive as a result of the difficulty in dissecting adhesions at this stage. Subsequently inadvertent bowel perforation may often occur, leading to renewed fistula formation.

If anastomotic failure amounts to half or more of the circumference of the anastomosis surrounded by an abscess, there is little likelihood of spontaneous closure and at some point in time salvage surgery is required. Breakdown of the anastomosis is however risky longer than one week after operation. Adequate drainage and diversion of the faecal stream are indicated at this point. In very low colo-rectal anastomoses disconnection should be postponed even longer because re-anastomosis is an enormous surgical challenge and fraught with potential complications [40]. When the abscess resulting from colo-rectal anastomotic leakage is limited, transanal drainage through the anastomotic defect may be considered, combined with deviation of the fecal stream by a double barrel colostomy or ileostomy.

In case of multi-locular abscesses and generalised peritonitis laparotomy and abdominal debridement is necessary followed by exteriorization or resection of the ruptured bowel or anastomosis.

Drainage

Although in some instances local surgical drainage may still be efficacious [42], there is a general tendency to aim for local ultrasound [43] or Ct-scan guided puncture drainage techniques [44, 45].

Local surgical drainage techniques are indicated when puncture techniques fail, the abscess contents are thick and not accessible to easy drainage *via* small bore drains although one report in the radiology literature claims that small bore drains are as efficacious as large bore drains [46]. Local drainage procedures are now more efficacious because Ct-scanning allows precise identification of the topography of the abscess. Small lateral incisions subcostally right or left, at Mc Burney's right or left, or *via* the 12th rib bed right or left can be performed to locally drain abscesses that cannot be drained adequately by image guided puncture.

There is some evidence that radiologic drainage procedures are efficacious, and that repeated drainage may increase efficacy of this approach [47-49]. Determinants of successful image guided puncture drainage are abscesses that are postoperative, not pancreatic, and not infected with yeast [48, 49].

Successful drainage of abscesses in Crohn's disease has been reported [50, 51]. This may be advantageous to diminish short-term infectious activity, and as preparation for definitive surgery. The nature of Crohn's diseases is such that once transmural inflammation has occurred leading to an abscess, the inflammatory process will eventually lead to scar formation and stricturing, necessitating surgical excision of the diseased bowel segment

[52]. Immunomodulatory therapy (infliximab, azathioprine, 6-mercaptopurine, methotrexate) has been reported to decrease the incidence of postoperative infectious complications in Crohn's disease [13].

Drains have not been proven to have prophylactic value, except in severe fecal appendicitis or peritonitis with well established and localised abscess cavities [53]. In this last situation the drain is of therapeutic rather than prophylactic use.

Conclusion

Knowledge of the risk factors involved in the development of postoperative infection may help to choose the timing and type of surgery that carries the least risks and to improve the condition of the patient by optimizing peri-operative conditions. Performing surgery during sepsis or in the presence of local infection carries the risk that an infection may result. Consequently all efforts should be directed towards diminishing inflammatory activity before operation. Similarly severe nutritional depletion should be treated if possible before operation. When the patient cannot survive post-operative infection due to depletion, immuno-suppression or organ failure, the least risky approach should be chosen. In general terms it is wise to adapt the surgical load and its risks to the ability of the patient to carry that load and to respond adequately to a renewed infectious challenge.

The choice to treat postoperative intra-abdominal infection locally or by full laparotomy depends on the time elapsed since operation. The earlier infectious symptoms become apparent, the more likely it is that they are serious and require re-laparotomy. After the first week infectious complications generally lead to walled-of abscesses and not to generalized peritonitis.

Modern advances in imaging techniques (ultrasound, Ct-scanning, MRI) have not only allowed precise delineation of the abscess(-es) but also percutaneous or local surgical drainage techniques, minimizing the necessity to perform laparotomies in a phase that laparotomy carries a substantial risk that the bowel will be inadvertently damaged.

References

1. von Meyenfeldt MF, Soeters PB. Risk factors for post-operative complications. *Br J Clin Pract Suppl* 1988; 63: 49-52.
2. Golub R, Golub RW, Cantu R Jr., Stein HD. A multivariate analysis of factors contributing to leakage of intestinal anastomoses. *J Am Coll Surg* 1997; 184: 364-72.
3. Tartter PI. Immunologic effects of blood transfusion. *Immunol Invest* 1995; 24: 277-88.
4. Mynster T, Nielsen HJ. The impact of storage time of transfused blood on postoperative infectious complications in rectal cancer surgery. Danish RANX05 Colorectal Cancer Study Group. *Scand J Gastroenterol* 2000; 35: 212-7.
5. Studley HO. Percentage weightloss, a basic indicator of surgical risk in patients with chronic peptic ulcer. *JAMA* 1936; 106: 458-60.

6. Klein S, Kinney J, Jeejeebhoy K, et al. Nutrition support in clinical practice: review of published data and recommendations for future research directions. National Institutes of Health, American Society for Parenteral and Enteral Nutrition, and American Society for Clinical Nutrition [see comments]. *JPEN J Parenter Enteral Nutr* 1997; 21: 133-56.
7. Ansari MZ, Collopy BT, Hart WG, Carson NJ, Chandraraj EJ. In-hospital mortality and associated complications after bowel surgery in Victorian public hospitals. *Aust N Z J Surg* 2000; 70: 6-10.
8. Clowes GH, Jr., Randall HT, Cha CJ. Amino acid and energy metabolism in septic and traumatized patients. *JPEN J Parenter Enteral Nutr* 1980; 4: 195-205.
9. Clowes GH, Jr., Hirsch E, George BC, Bigatello LM, Mazuski JE, Villee CA, Jr. Survival from sepsis. The significance of altered protein metabolism regulated by proteolysis inducing factor, the circulating cleavage product of interleukin-1. *Ann Surg* 1985; 202: 446-58.
10. Puggioni A, Wong LL. A metaanalysis of laparoscopic cholecystectomy in patients with cirrhosis. *J Am Coll Surg* 2003; 197: 921-6.
11. Sorensen LT, Jorgensen T, Kirkeby LT, Skovdal J, Vennits B, Wille-Jorgensen P. Smoking and alcohol abuse are major risk factors for anastomotic leakage in colorectal surgery. *Br J Surg* 1999; 86: 927-31.
12. Kasperk R, Philipps B, Vahrmeyer M, Willis S, Schumpelick V. [Risk factors for anastomosis dehiscence after very deep colorectal and coloanal anastomosis]. *Chirurg* 2000; 71: 1365-9.
13. Tay GS, Binion DG, Eastwood D, Otterson MF. Multivariate analysis suggests improved perioperative outcome in Crohn's disease patients receiving immunomodulator therapy after segmental resection and/or strictureplasty. *Surgery* 2003; 134: 565-72; discussion 72-3.
14. Linder MM, Wacha H, Feldmann U, Wesch G, Streifensand RA, Gundlach E. [The Mannheim peritonitis index. An instrument for the intraoperative prognosis of peritonitis]. *Chirurg* 1987; 58: 84-92.
15. Schirrmacher E, Seifert J. [The Mannheim Peritonitis Index. Its reliability for the assessment of prognosis in peritonitis patients]. *Fortschr Med* 1988; 106: 454-6.
16. Grunau G, Heemken R, Hau T. Predictors of outcome in patients with postoperative intra-abdominal infection. *Eur J Surg* 1996; 162: 619-25.
17. Schilling MK, Maurer CA, Kollmar O, Buchler MW. Primary vs. secondary anastomosis after sigmoid colon resection for perforated diverticulitis (Hinchey Stage III and IV): a prospective outcome and cost analysis. *Dis Colon Rectum* 2001; 44: 699-703; discussion -5.
18. Hansen O, Graupe F, Stock W. [Prognostic factors in perforating diverticulitis of the large intestine]. *Chirurg* 1998; 69: 443-9.
19. Schwartz SR, Yueh B, Maynard C, Daley J, Henderson W, Khuri SF. Predictors of wound complications after laryngectomy: A study of over 2,000 patients. *Otolaryngol Head Neck Surg* 2004; 131: 61-8.
20. Kirkpatrick AW, Baxter KA, Simons RK, Germann E, Lucas CE, Ledgerwood AM. Intra-abdominal complications after surgical repair of small bowel injuries: an international review. *J Trauma* 2003; 55: 399-406.
21. Beck DE, Cohen Z, Fleshman JW, Kaufman HS, van Goor H, Wolff BG. A prospective, randomized, multicenter, controlled study of the safety of Seprafilm adhesion barrier in abdominopelvic surgery of the intestine. *Dis Colon Rectum* 2003; 46: 1310-9.
22. Pedersen AG, Petersen OB, Wara P, Ronning H, Qvist N, Laurberg S. Randomized clinical trial of laparoscopic versus open appendicectomy. *Br J Surg* 2001; 88: 200-5.
23. Horwitz JR, Custer MD, May BH, Mehall JR, Lally KP. Should laparoscopic appendectomy be avoided for complicated appendicitis in children? *J Pediatr Surg* 1997; 32: 1601-3.
24. Katkhouda N, Friedlander MH, Grant SW, et al. Intraabdominal abscess rate after laparoscopic appendectomy. *Am J Surg* 2000; 180: 456-9; discussion 60-1.
25. Andersen BR, Kallehave FL, Andersen HK. Antibiotics versus placebo for prevention of postoperative infection after appendicectomy. *Cochrane Database Syst Rev* 2003 (2): CD001439.

26. Klein. Nutrition support in clinical practice: review of published data and recommendations for future research directions. *Clin Nutr* 1997; 19: 193-218.
27. Heyland DK, Dhaliwal R, Drover JW, Gramlich L, Dodek P. Canadian clinical practice guidelines for nutrition support in mechanically ventilated, critically ill adult patients. *JPEN J Parenter Enteral Nutr* 2003; 27: 355-73.
28. Heyland DK, Novak F, Drover JW, Jain M, Su X, Suchner U. Should immunonutrition become routine in critically ill patients? A systematic review of the evidence. *JAMA* 2001; 286: 944-53.
29. Zmora O, Mahajna A, Bar-Zakai B, et al. Colon and rectal surgery without mechanical bowel preparation: a randomized prospective trial. *Ann Surg* 2003; 237: 363-7.
30. Burke P, Mealy K, Gillen P, Joyce W, Traynor O, Hyland J. Requirement for bowel preparation in colorectal surgery. *Br J Surg* 1994; 81: 907-10.
31. Cohn SM, Giannotti G, Ong AW, et al. Prospective randomized trial of two wound management strategies for dirty abdominal wounds. *Ann Surg* 2001; 233: 409-13.
32. Luna-Perez P, Rodriguez-Ramirez S, Gonzalez-Macouzet J, Rodriguez-Coria DF. [Treatment of anastomotic leakage following low anterior resection for rectal adenocarcinoma]. *Rev Invest Clin* 1999; 51: 23-9.
33. Marik PE, Zaloga GP. Hypothermia and cytokines in septic shock. Norasept II Study Investigators. North American study of the safety and efficacy of murine monoclonal antibody to tumor necrosis factor for the treatment of septic shock. *Intens Care Med* 2000; 26: 716-21.
34. Bearcroft PW, Miles KA. Leucocyte scintigraphy or computed tomography for the febrile post-operative patient? *Eur J Radiol* 1996; 23: 126-9.
35. Palestro CJ, Love C, Tronco GG, Tomas MB. Role of radionuclide imaging in the diagnosis of postoperative infection. *Radiographics* 2000; 20: 1649-60; discussion 60-3.
36. Tsai SC, Chao TH, Lin WY, Wang SJ. Abdominal abscesses in patients having surgery: an application of Ga-67 scintigraphic and computed tomographic scanning. *Clin Nucl Med* 2001; 26: 761-4.
37. Lin WY, Chao TH, Wang SJ. Clinical features and gallium scan in the detection of post-surgical infection in the elderly. *Eur J Nucl Med Mol Imaging* 2002; 29: 371-5.
38. Ketai L, Washington T, Allen T, Rael J. Is the stat Gram stain helpful during percutaneous image-guided fluid drainage? *Acad Radiol* 2000; 7: 228-31.
39. Hardwick RH, Taylor A, Thompson MH, Jones E, Roe AM. Association between Streptococcus milleri and abscess formation after appendicitis. *Ann R Coll Surg Engl* 2000; 82: 24-6.
40. Parc Y, Frileux P, Schmitt G, Dehni N, Ollivier JM, Parc R. Management of postoperative peritonitis after anterior resection: experience from a referral intensive care unit. *Dis Colon Rectum* 2000; 43: 579-87; discussion 87-9.
41. Soeters PB, de Zoete JP, Dejong CH, Williams NS, Baeten CG. Colorectal surgery and anastomotic leakage. *Dig Surg* 2002; 19: 150-5.
42. Spain DA, Martin RC, Carrillo EH, Polk HC, Jr. Twelfth rib resection. Preferred therapy for subphrenic abscess in selected surgical patients. *Arch Surg* 1997; 132: 1203-6.
43. Civardi G, Di Candio G, Giorgio A, et al. Ultrasound guided percutaneous drainage of abdominal abscesses in the hands of the clinician: a multicenter Italian study. *Eur J Ultrasound* 1998; 8: 91-9.
44. Lee MJ. Non-traumatic abdominal emergencies: imaging and intervention in sepsis. *Eur Radiol* 2002; 12: 2172-9.
45. Men S, Akhan O, Koroglu M. Percutaneous drainage of abdominal abcess. *Eur J Radiol* 2002; 43: 204-18.
46. Rothlin MA, Schob O, Klotz H, Candinas D, Largiader F. Percutaneous drainage of abdominal abscesses: are large-bore catheters necessary? *Eur J Surg* 1998; 164: 419-24.
47. Bufalari A, Giustozzi G, Moggi L. Postoperative intraabdominal abscesses: percutaneous versus surgical treatment. *Acta Chir Belg* 1996; 96: 197-200.
48. Cinat ME, Wilson SE, Din AM. Determinants for successful percutaneous image-guided drainage of intra-abdominal abscess. *Arch Surg* 2002; 137: 845-9.

49. Gervais DA, Ho CH, O'Neill MJ, Arellano RS, Hahn PF, Mueller PR. Recurrent abdominal and pelvic abscesses: incidence, results of repeated percutaneous drainage, and underlying causes in 956 drainages. *AJR Am J Roentgenol* 2004; 182: 463-6.
50. Ayuk P, Williams N, Scott NA, Nicholson DA, Irving MH. Management of intra-abdominal abscesses in Crohn's disease. *Ann R Coll Surg Engl* 1996; 78: 5-10.
51. Sahai A, Belair M, Gianfelice D, Cote S, Gratton J, Lahaie R. Percutaneous drainage of intra-abdominal abscesses in Crohn's disease: short and long-term outcome. *Am J Gastroenterol* 1997; 92: 275-8.
52. Gervais DA, Hahn PF, O'Neill MJ, Mueller PR. Percutaneous abscess drainage in Crohn disease: technical success and short- and long-term outcomes during 14 years. *Radiology* 2002; 222: 645-51.
53. Kokoska ER, Silen ML, Tracy TF, Jr., Dillon PA, Cradock TV, Weber TR. Perforated appendicitis in children: risk factors for the development of complications. *Surgery* 1998; 124: 619-25; discussion 25-6.

VI

Transferring the pediatric patient to "adult" care

Celiac disease in children and adolescents

Yigael Finkel

Karolinska Institute, Stockholm, Sweden

Celiac disease is a disorder induced by wheat, rye, and barley proteins, and its classic form is characterized in children by malabsorption and failure to thrive. During the past two decades, however, the clinical picture of the disease has changed to include milder forms, thus resulting in an upward shift of the age at diagnosis. Screening for active celiac disease use serum autoantibodies, and in most centres only tissue transglutaminase antibodies are used [1]. The screeing for celiac disease in children usually focuses on patients with mild gastrointestinal symptoms, isolated iron deficiency, atypical or extraintestinal manifestations of autoimmune diseases or on the first-degree relatives of affected patients. Screening programs within populations indicate that the disease is underdiagnosed.

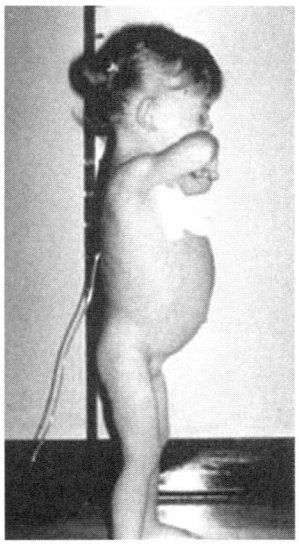

Figure 1. Typical presentation of celiac disease in a young child.

The presence of serum tissue transglutaminase and endomysial autoantibodies is predictive of small-bowel abnormalities indicative of celiac disease. There is a good correlation between autoantibody positivity and specific HLA haplotypes. A recent population based study estimate that the prevalence of celiac disease among Finnish schoolchildren is at least 1 case in 99 children [2].

Celiac disease is characterized by intestinal villus atrophy and malabsorption. The disease is dependent on the ingestion of prolamins derived from wheat, barley, or rye proteins, which are characterized by their high content in glutamine (35%) and proline (20%).

Approximately 90% of patients with celiac disease carry the HLA-DQ2 heterodimer encoded by the HLA-DQA1*05 and DQB1*02 genes.

Most of the remaining 10% of patients have the HLA-DR4-DQ8 haplotype.

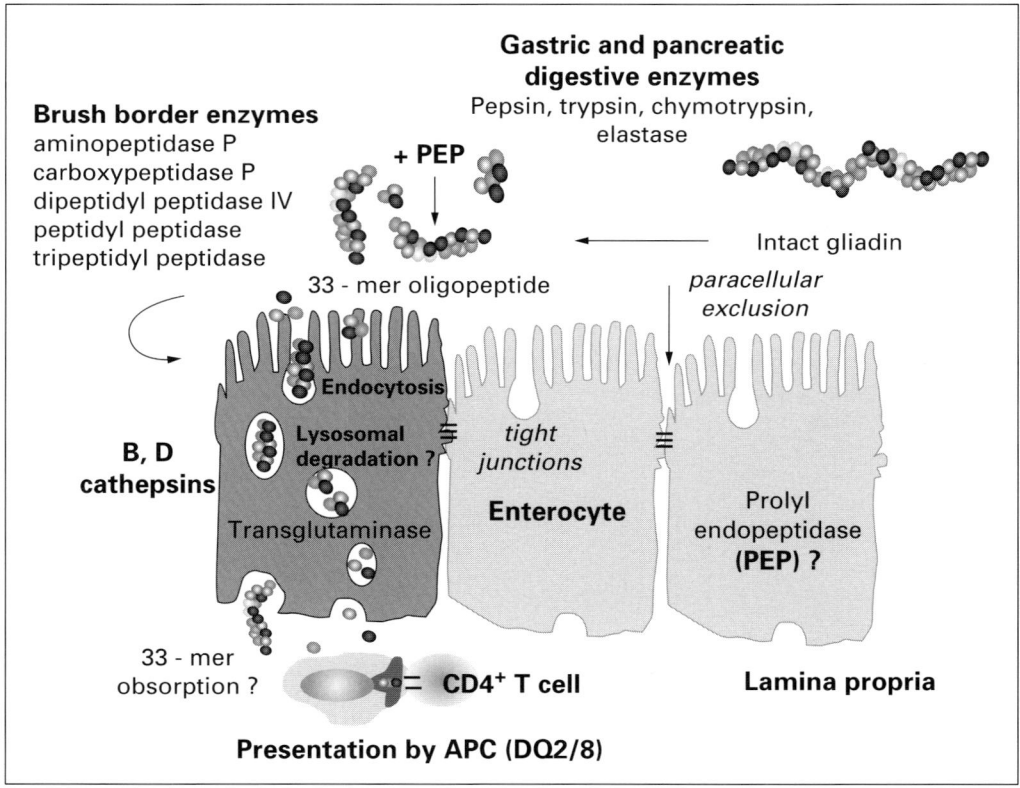

Figure 2. The immune reaction to gliadin: a 33-mer peptide derived from gliadin is resistant to the degradation by luminal digestive enzymes and peptidases of the brush border membrane. This peptide also efficiently stimulates the proliferation of intestinal CD4+ T cells, after treatment with transglutaminase, in celiac patients [3]. This figure appears in [4].

Celiac disease is treated with gluten-free diet. During the last years there have been reports on the use of oat in the gluten-free diet of celiac patients, with a few reported cases of side-effects in adult celiac patients during follow up.

The compliance with gluten-free diet is expensive. The Swedish Consumer Agency has calculated that a gluten-free is approximately 20% more expensive that a regular diet. Complying with gluten-free diet may affect normal everyday social life and spare time activities. Most children are diagnosed at an age when they cannot be expected to psychologically ally to comply with gluten-free diet. It is therefore more a rule than an exception that teen-agers openly or secretely wish to test or actively go about to test the diagnosis.

An Italian study on compliance with gluten-free diet in adolescents with screening-detected celiac disease showed that after five years of treatment, 22 patients with celiac disease, diagnosed by means of serologic mass screening, showed a lower compliance with a gluten-free diet and frequent positivity of serum anti-endomysium antibodies (32%) in comparison with a group of 22 age-matched patients diagnosed because of "typical" symptoms during childhood [5].

Similarly in a study of 123 patients with celiac disease, diagnosed in the first three years of life and reevaluated during the teenage period showed that 65% of these adolescents were adhering to a strict gluten free diet, 11% were on a gluten free diet but with occasional gluten intake, and 24% were on a gluten containing diet. Clinical symptoms occurred more frequently in patients on a gluten containing diet, but not in patients on a semi-strict diet. Occasional intake of small amounts (0.06-2 g/day) of gluten did not produce increased concentrations of antigliadin antibodies but resulted in histopathological changes in small bowel biopsies such as appreciably increased crypt epithelial volume and expanded crypt intraepithelial lymphocyte population [6].

References

1. Korponay-Szabo IR, Sulkanen S, Halttunen T, Maurano F, Rossi M, Mazzarella G, Laurila K, Troncone R, Maki M. Tissue transglutaminase is the target in both rodent and primate tissues for celiac disease-specific autoantibodies. *J Pediatr Gastroenterol Nutr* 2000; 31: 520-7.
2. Maki M, Mustalahti K, Kokkonen J, Kulmala P, Haapalahti M, Karttunen T, Ilonen J, Laurila K, Dahlbom I, Hansson T, Hopfl P, Knip M. Prevalence of Celiac disease among children in Finland. *N Engl J Med* 2003; 348: 2517-24.
3. Shan L, Molberg O, Parrot I, Hausch F, Filiz F, Gray GM, Sollid LM, Khosla C. Structural basis for gluten intolerance in celiac sprue. *Science* 2002; 297: 2275-9.
4. Cerf-Bensussan N, Heyman M. *J Pediatr Gastroenterol Nutr* 2003; 36: 585-6.
5. Fabiani E, Taccari LM, Ratsch IM, Di Giuseppe S, Coppa GV, Catassi C. Compliance with gluten-free diet in adolescents with screening-detected celiac disease: a 5-year follow-up study. *J Pediatr* 2000; 136: 841-3.
6. Mayer M, Greco L, Troncone R, Auricchio S, Marsh MN. Compliance of adolescents with coeliac disease with a gluten free diet. *Gut* 1991; 32: 881-5.

New Developments in the Management of Benign GI Disorders.
D.J. Gouma, G.J. Krejs, G.N. Tytgat, Y. Finkel, eds. John Libbey Eurotext, Paris © 2004, pp. 175-180.

Celiac disease from childhood to adulthood

H. Vogelsang

Department of Internal Medicine IV, Division of Gastroenterology and Hepatology, General Hospital of Vienna, Waehringer Guertel, Vienna, Austria

It is well known that it was Samuel Gee in 1888 [1] who published a first detailed description in modern times of what he calls the celiac affection: "There is a kind of chronic indigestion which is met in persons of all ages; yet it is especially found to affect the children between one and five years old... Signs of the disease are yielded by the faeces, being loose but not watery, bulky and pale...". Already this statement described celiac disease (CD) as a disease affecting all ages although it was especially recognized in young children. Thus celiac disease had a similar story in Austria. Primarily young patients with celiac disease were diagnosed at the pediatric departments with an increasing frequency of celiac diagnosis also in "adult" internal departments from 1990 on (Vogelsang, *Granditsch* 2001, unpublished results, *figure 1*). By the help of new serological tests as endomysial antibodies and recently tissue transglutaminase antibodies an increased prevalence of celiac disease was also found in the adult population. During the last years celiac disease was found much more frequently in the specialized outdoor ambulance for adults than in the pediatric special ambulance. The legislative situation in Austria determines that the pediatrician could be responsible for patients from 0-19 years while internal medicines usually take care of patients from 15 years of age.

Prevalence

Overall the prevalence of celiac disease has augmented from 1 of 1,000 healthy people [2] to 1 of 100 healthy people in recent studies [3-5]. A rapid increase of newly diagnosed patients had taken place because of the newer screening tests and better understanding of disease. Especially silent celiac disease without any typical or predominant symptoms from the abdomen has developed as the leading form of celiac disease affecting more than 2/3 of newly diagnosed patients [6]. This increase of silent celiac disease patients has been found as well in children as in adults [3, 6]. The onset of disease is in about half of

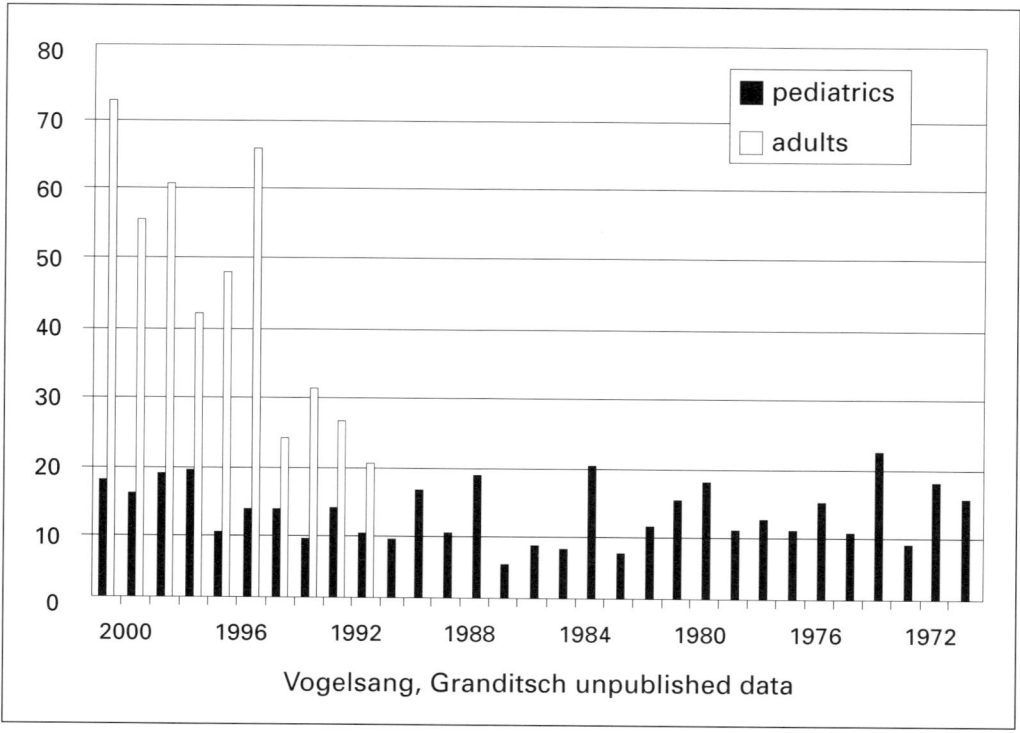

Figure 1. New patients with celiac disease at the pediatric and the "adult" internal department 1972-2000.

the patients in the childhood and about half (more than 50%) in the adulthood – already published more than ten years ago [7]. The median age at diagnosis of children is below 10 years –and has been delayed during the last years – and of adults the age of 40. Patients with CD show a more than 95% prevalence of two HLA class II types [8] especially of HLA DQ2 and minor of HLA DQ8 which is of high importance for the pathogenesis of CD. The reason for late onset celiac disease, however, could be different HLA class I traits. Our group has found that patients with onset in adulthood more often show the HLA A1 B8 Cw7 type [9].

Diagnosis

In the meantime, there are three different consensus papers on the diagnosis of celiac disease – the older and the newer ESPGAN-criteria [10] and now the Amsterdam-criteria [11]. The last international consensus conference in Amsterdam decided that one typical small bowel biopsy showing villous atrophy confirmed by resolution of symptoms – usually followed by normalization of previous abnormal serology tests – under gluten free diet is diagnostic for celiac disease. While pediatricians still use capsules for small bowel biopsies, adult patients are now routinely biopsied from the distal duodenum during upper

GI-endoscopy [12]. A standardized report scheme for pathologists is challenged to classify the biopsies of celiac patients [13]. The so-called modified criteria according to MARSH are identifying celiac disease from MARSH 3a, 3b to 3c. MARSH 0, MARSH 1 and 2 are not sufficient for diagnosis of celiac disease. The use of serological tests as endomysial antibodies [14] and tissue transglutaminase antibodies [15] for screening are now recommended for all ages although antigliadin antibodies could be of some significance in children with less than two yeas of age.

The recovery of small bowel celiac lesions is much quicker in children than in adults, as more 90% of celiac children show complete recovery of duodenal or jejunal mucosa in comparison to only about 65% of adult celiac patients after two years of diet [16]. Therefore control biopsies in adults should not be done – if necessary at all – earlier than after two years under gluten free diet.

Follow-up

There are several differences in the management of disease as already mentioned: biopsies are taken by capsules often in children and by endoscopy in adults and also concerning the diet counseling which is done in children with CD as well to the patients themselves as to their parents. In adults, of course, the diet counseling is mainly done to the patients themselves. There is a big problem in follow-up of patients under gluten free diet, especially in adolescents. Many young people try to leave the gluten free diet and continue on a free diet because only a few of them are experiencing symptoms. Therefore, there is a need for continuous follow-ups at specialized outdoor ambulances or gastroenterologists. Growing up patients should be transferred to the adult departments together with their often long medical records [17].

A continuous follow-up of these adolescents and later of the adults is recommended to achieve a complete adherence to the diet and to avoid complications [18]. An Italian study presented at DDW 2004 in New Orleans [19] showed in 215 grown-ups (median age 21 years, with celiac disease diagnosed in childhood) that celiac disease could not be confirmed in 5% of patients. Even 34% of 110 patients on a primarily strict gluten free diet showed regular gluten ingestion at the interview and 80% of them showed villous atrophy. Out of the 44% on free diet 15 of 85 showed dental enamel defects and one patient (19 years) even died due to enteropathy associated T-cell lymphoma. There should be a close cooperation of pediatric and adult departments in order to follow-up the growing children with celiac disease [17].

Complications

There are some differences also in the course of disease. The complications of celiac disease [12] are rare in children; however there are several severe ones in adult patients: miscarriages, autoimmune diseases, fractures and lymphoma; these complications take place only in patients with late diagnosis or not adhering to gluten free diet.

The appearance of dermatitis herpetiformis Duhring is very rarely reported in children but in about 10% of adults [20]. Refractory celiac disease is nearly unknown in children but concerns about 2% (our unpublished data) of the adults [21]. Enteropathy associated T-cell lymphoma is only a problem of about 0.03% of adult celiac patients, especially patients diagnosed after 50 years of age [22, 23]. There is a frequent association with various autoimmune diseases in adults [24]; only some children suffer from diabetes mellitus [25] or thyroid diseases Osteoporosis a mainly a problem of adults before starting gluten free diet and never a problem to children [26, 27], although children with CD might suffer from decreased height growth [28].

As about 10-15% of patients with celiac disease have relatives which are also affected by celiac disease [29], a screening of the first degree relatives should be done. Relatives younger than 15 years may be screened by the pediatric department and those of more than 15 years of age at the internal medicine department.

In addition, there is a big field also for scientific cooperation to test the differences of population because of genetic background of disease, diagnosis and course of disease.

There are recent studies showing high prevalence of celiac disease in children. An English study comprising 5,470 children at the age of 7.5 years showed positive endomysial and tissue transglutaminase antibodies in about 1% of patients [30]. These patients were shorter, had less weight and more often suffered from diarrhea (about 50% vs 30% in negative controls). This prevalence is similar to that of celiac disease in the whole population (1%). Therefore, all patients with celiac disease could be already diagnosed at the age of 7 years if a screening would be done...

There are some other problems in the management of children or adolescents with celiac disease. Children might have higher sensitivity to gliadin and oats [31] although not proven [32].

Conclusion

A close cooperation between pediatric and adult department is important. This secures the transfer of medical records and helps to get a consensus on diagnosis and treatment of celiac patients independent of their age. There is a need for motivation of adolescents to stick to gluten free diet strictly which could only be achieved by cooperation of both departments. On the other side there is a big chance of scientific collaboration of the two departments, especially with respect to the pathogenesis of the disease.

References

1. Gee S. On the celiac affection. *St. Bart Hosp Rep* 1890; 24: 17-20.
2. Maki M, Kallonen K, Lahdeaho ML, Visakorpi JK. Changing pattern of childhood coeliac disease in Finland. *Acta Paediatr Scand* 1988; 77: 408-12.

3. Korponay-Szabo IR, Kovacs JB, Czinner A, Goracz G, Vamos A, Szabo T. High prevalence of silent celiac disease in preschool children screened with IgA/IgG antiendomysium antibodies. *J Pediatr Gastroenterol Nutr* 1999; 28: 26-30.
4. Maki M, Mustalahti K, Kokkonen J, Kulmala P, Haapalahti M, Karttunen T, Ilonen J, Laurila K, Dahlbom I, Hansson T, Hopfl P, Knip M. Prevalence of Celiac disease among children in Finland. *N Engl J Med* 2003; 348: 2517-24.
5. Fasano A, Berti I, Gerarduzzi T, Not T, Colletti RB, Drago S, Elitsur Y, Green PH, Guandalini S, Hill ID, Pietzak M, Ventura A, Thorpe M, Kryszak D, Fornaroli F, Wasserman SS, Murray JA, Horvath K. Prevalence of celiac disease in at-risk and not-at-risk groups in the United States: a large multicenter study. *Arch Intern Med* 2003; 163: 286-92.
6. Bottaro G, Cataldo F, Rotolo N, Spina M, Corazza GR. The clinical pattern of subclinical/silent celiac disease: an analysis on 1,026 consecutive cases. *Am J Gastroenterol* 1999; 94: 691-6.
7. Jansen TLTA, Mulder CJJ, Karssen PHZ, Wagenaar CJJ. Epidemiological survey of the Dutch Coeliac Disease Society: an update 1992. *Eur J Gastroenterol Hepatol* 1993; 5: 73-8.
8. Maki M, Mustalahti K, Kokkonen J, Kulmala P, Haapalahti M, Karttunen T, Ilonen J, Laurila K, Dahlbom I, Hansson T, Hopfl P, Knip M. Prevalence of Celiac disease among children in Finland. *N Engl J Med* 2003; 348: 2517-24.
9. Vogelsang H, Panzer S, Mayr WR, Granditsch G, Fischer GF. Distribution of HLA class I alleles differs in celiac disease patients according to age of onset. *Dig Dis Sci* 2003; 48: 611.
10. Walker-Smith JA, Guandalini S, Schmitz J, Shmerling DH, Visakorpi JK. Revised criteria for diagnosis of coeliac disease. *Arch Dis Child* 1990; 65: 909-11.
11. When is a coeliac a coeliac? Report of a working group of the United European Gastroenterology Week in Amsterdam. *Gut* 2001.
12. Vogelsang H, Propst A, Dragosics B, Granditsch G. Working Group for Chronic Inflammatory Bowel Diseases of the Austrian Society of Gastroenterology and Hepatology. [Diagnosis and therapy of celiac disease in adolescence and adulthood]. *Z Gastroenterol* 2002; 40: I-VII.
13. Oberhuber G, Granditsch G, Vogelsang H. The histopathology of coeliac disease: time for a standardized report scheme for pathologists. *Eur J Gastroenterol Hepatol* 1999; 11: 1185-94. Review.
14. Vogelsang H, Genser D, Wyatt J, Lochs H, Ferenci P, Granditsch G, Penner E. Screening for celiac disease: a prospective study on the value of noninvasive tests. *Am J Gastroenterol* 1995; 90: 394-8.
15. Burgin-Wolff A, Dahlbom I, Hadziselimovic F, Petersson CJ. Antibodies against human tissue transglutaminase and endomysium in diagnosing and monitoring coeliac disease. *Scand J Gastroenterol* 2002; 37: 685-91.
16. Wahab PJ, Meijer JW, Mulder CJ. Histologic follow-up of people with celiac disease on a gluten-free diet: slow and incomplete recovery. *Am J Clin Pathol* 2002; 118: 459-63.
17. Ciclitira PJ, Moodie SJ. Transition of care between paediatric and adult gastroenterology. Coeliac Disease. *Best Pract Res Clin Gastroenterol* 2003; 17: 181-95. Review.
18. Fabiani E, Taccari LM, Ratsch IM, Di Giuseppe S, Coppa GV, Catassi C. Compliance with gluten-free diet in adolescents with screening-detected celiac disease: a 5-year follow-up study. *J Pediatr* 2000; 136: 841-3.
19. Ciacci C, Iovino P, Amoruso D, Siniscalchi M, Tortura R, Di Gilio A, Mazzacca G. Celiac children grow up. *Gastroenterology* 2004: 5.
20. Fry L. Dermatitis herpetiformis: problems, progress and prospects. *Eur J Dermatol* 2002; 12: 523-31. Review.
21. Culliford AN, Green PH. Refractory sprue. *Curr Gastroenterol Rep* 2003; 5: 373-8. Review.
22. Catassi C, Fabiani E, Corrao G, Barbato M, De Renzo A, Carella AM, Gabrielli A, Leoni P, Carroccio A, Baldassarre M, Bertolani P, Caramaschi P, Sozzi M, Guariso G, Volta U, Corazza GR. Italian Working Group on Coeliac Disease and Non-Hodgkin's-Lymphoma. Risk of non-Hodgkin lymphoma in celiac disease. *JAMA* 2002; 287: 1413-9.

23. Hoffmann M, Vogelsang H, Kletter K, Zettinig G, Chott A, Raderer M. 18F-fluoro-deoxy-glucose positron emission tomography (18F-FDG-PET) for assessment of enteropathy-type T cell lymphoma. *Gut* 2003; 52: 347-51.
24. Ventura A, Magazzu G, Greco L. Duration of exposure to gluten and risk for autoimmune disorders in patients with celiac disease. SIGEP Study Group for Autoimmune Disorders in Celiac Disease. *Gastroenterology* 1999; 117: 297-303.
25. Crone J, Rami B, Huber WD, Granditsch G, Schober E. Prevalence of celiac disease and follow-up of EMA in children and adolescents with type 1 diabetes mellitus. *J Pediatr Gastroenterol Nutr* 2003; 37: 67-71.
26. West J, Logan RF, Card TR, Smith C, Hubbard R. Fracture risk in people with celiac disease: a population-based cohort study. *Gastroenterology* 2003; 125: 429-36.
27. Kemppainen T, Kroger H, Janatuinen E, Arnala I, Lamberg-Allardt C, Karkkainen M, Kosma VM, Julkunen R, Jurvelin J, Alhava E, Uusitupa M. Bone recovery after a gluten-free diet: a 5-year follow-up study. *Bone* 1999; 25: 355-60.
28. Sdepanian VL, de Miranda Carvalho CN, de Morais MB, Colugnati FA, Fagundes-Neto U. Bone mineral density of the lumbar spine in children and adolescents with celiac disease on a gluten-free diet in Sao Paulo, Brazil. *J Pediatr Gastroenterol Nutr* 2003; 37: 571-6.
29. Vogelsang H, Wyatt J, Penner E, Lochs H. Screening for celiac disease in first-degree relatives of patients with celiac disease by lactulose/mannitol test. *Am J Gastroenterol* 1995; 90: 1838-42.
30. Bingley PJ, Williams AJ, Norcross AJ, Unsworth DJ, Lock RJ, Ness AR, Jones RW. Avon Longitudinal Study of Parents and Children Study Team. Undiagnosed coeliac disease at age seven: population based prospective birth cohort study. *Br Med J* 2004; 328: 322-3.
31. Janatuinen EK, Kemppainen TA, Julkunen RJ, Kosma VM, Maki M, Heikkinen M, Uusitupa MI. No harm from five year ingestion of oats in coeliac disease. *Gut* 2002; 50: 332-5.
32. Hogberg L, Laurin P, Falth-Magnusson K, Grant C, Grodzinsky E, Jansson G, Ascher H, Browaldh L, Hammersjo JA, Lindberg E, Myrdal U, Stenhammar L. Oats to children with newly diagnosed coeliac disease: a randomised double blind study. *Gut* 2004; 53: 649-54.

Transition of the liver transplant recipient to adult care

D.A. Kelly

The Liver Unit, Birmingham Children's Hospital, Birmingham, United Kingdom

The survival rate for child and adolescent recipients of liver transplantation is 80% over 15 years. The challenge of developing transitional care for these young people is based on effective collaboration at the paediatric-adult interface and is a major challenge for paediatric and adult providers alike in the 21st century.

What is transition?

Transition has been defined, as "a multi-faceted, active process that attends to the medical, psychosocial and educational/vocational needs of adolescents as they move from child to adult centred care" [1]. The aims of transition are:

(i) to provide high quality, co-ordinated, uninterrupted healthcare which is patient-centred, age and developmentally appropriate, culturally competent, flexible, responsive and comprehensive;

(ii) to promote skills in communication, decision-making, assertiveness, self-care and self-advocacy;

(iii) to enhance sense of control and interdependence in healthcare;

(iv) to maximize life-long functioning and potential.

Many adult physicians will not be familiar with these "new" diseases as these patients usually died during childhood, *e.g.* inborn errors of metabolism prior to effective therapy or the development of transplantation. Information from adult physicians regarding long-term outcome data is vital for counselling young people with these conditions by their paediatric colleagues.

Transitional care acknowledges the reciprocal influences of adolescent bio-psychosocial development and the underlying chronic illness and transplantation. As well as transitioning from paediatric to adult care, adolescents who have undergone liver transplantation have also made a transition from a familiar or well-known end-stage disease to a different chronic condition. They may still have an uncertain future, remain dependent on a medical team, have to adjust to complex medication regimes, accept changes in their external appearance and adjust to significant lifestyle changes. They may continue to require periods of hospitalisation, and even further surgery.

Chronic illness may affect physical development during adolescence, *e.g.* delayed sexual maturation and physical growth. Physical growth in turn can affect the pharmacokinetics of drugs, *e.g.* increased sensitivity to corticosteroid toxicity at puberty. Cognitive development is driven by increasing myelination and maturation of the central nervous system during adolescence, and results in the development of more adult-like abstract thinking and a more complete personal identity. This can be affected by drug side effects, school side effects, pain, fatigue, etc. The stage of cognitive development is important in planning health and disease education for such young people as well as their involvement in decision-making and self-care. In contrast to the biological and cognitive changes, which are fairly universal, the psychosocial changes of adolescence are largely culturally determined. In Western cultures, the social "tasks" of adolescence are concerned with establishing relationships outside the family, achieving independence from parents and establishing financial (*i.e.* vocational) independence. These processes are outlined in *table I*.

Conversely, the imperatives of adolescent development (the search for identity and independence, immature abstract thinking, etc.) may make chronic illness management problematic through poor adherence to medical regimens and "risky" health behaviours.

Table I. Main tasks of adolescence

1. To consolidate his/her identity
2. To establish relationships outside the family
3. To achieve independence from parents
4. To find a vocation

The differences between paediatric and adult health care

There are disease-specific differences in that paediatric liver transplant recipients themselves differ from their adult counterparts in terms of age, primary diagnoses, type of graft, donor population, post-transplant complications in addition to a longer potential life span in which to develop complications, *e.g.* recurrent disease, osteoporosis, atherosclerosis, renal failure, post-transplant malignancies [2].

- **Growth and development:** the bidirectional influences of a chronic illness and adolescent development (physical, cognitive and psychosocial) need to be anticipated and addressed by the multidisciplinary transplant teams. Evidence from other chronic illnesses suggests that both paediatricians and adult physicians are poor at monitoring growth and pubertal development in chronic illness, and continued attention is required to growth in chronic illness well into the early twenties especially when there has been growth retardation due to the primary disease [3]. Conversely, as young people become older adults, health providers need to be skilled at age appropriate management for this age-group, *i.e.* adult medicine rather than paediatric medicine.

- **Consultation dynamics :** the paternalistic triangular model that is characteristic of paediatric care with parent, professional and child, moves through various models during adolescence until the horizontal adult relationship of patient and professional is achieved. Communication and counselling skills are important aspects of training for those working with young people in this age group, and there is evidence from randomised trials that these skills can be learned [4].

- **Communication skills :** acquiring mastery of such consultations requires communication skills and strategies, which may vary depending on the subject matter and circumstance as well as the respective stage of adolescent development, etc.

As they mature, young people normally develop from using emotional strategies (such as wishful thinking or resignation) to problem-solving strategies. Chronic illness can interfere with this development or cause the adolescent to regress in this respect. Unpredictable diseases often tend to encourage the use of emotion-focused coping strategies. Emotion-based coping strategies have been related to self-reports of depression, anxiety and substance abuse in adolescents whereas when a problem-based approach is used, mothers and young people report fewer emotional and behaviour problems [9].

When should transition take place?

The essence of transitional care is that it ideally starts early, with promotion of resilience and self-determination in the young person, whatever their age, and their families. There is no single or arbitrary milestone that heralds transition readiness in an individual patient and their parent(s). In keeping with the concept of transition being a process, there is no age cut-off for the end of transition or the event of transfer to adult care. The essence of timing in all aspects of transition is that of flexibility. Timing of events within the transitional process will depend on many variables and must be individualized for each patient *(table II)*. Any plan for transition and transfer should be regularly reviewed particularly in the context of an unpredictable chronic condition as needs will change. Ideally the preparation should start well before the process needs to begin. Discussion and preparation for transition needs relative disease remission (if possible) and transfer should definitely not be implemented during an "active" phase of their disease.

Who is involved in transition?

The key player in the process of transition is the young person his/herself. Family connectedness, family role models, family concern for the well-being of the child and autonomy at home are all factors identified that foster resilience in children and should be encouraged

Table II. Timing of transition and transfer

- Chronological age
- Maturity
- Current medical status
- Adherence to therapy
- Independence in healthcare
- Preparation
- Readiness of the young person
- Availability of an appropriate adult specialist

and affirmed [5], especially during adolescence and transition. Conversely, lack of parental support at this time has been associated with negative outcomes eg greater non-adherence to medication [6].

Just as the young person with a chronic condition is negotiating the tasks and transitions detailed above, their parent(s) is also having to negotiate the transition of being a parent of a dependent child with a chronic illness to a parent of an independent young adult with a chronic illness – not always easy. Parents therefore also need a preparation period for transition and transfer. Programmes should support parents in developing an understanding of adolescent development in the context of chronic illness, their own important, dynamic role in the process, advice renegotiation of boundaries and the resources available both within the hospital and the local community. Parents can be helped to encourage involvement of their son/daughter in decision-making from an early age, to ensure attainment of functional living skills and development of autonomy and self-advocacy skills.

Key players in transition include an identified health professional for each young person, the multidisciplinary transplant team in both the paediatric and adult transplant units and the primary health care team. Health professionals cannot work in isolation from the other professionals and networks that impact young people with chronic conditions and hence other key players include members of the education services (including careers and vocational rehabilitation), social services and voluntary organizations who may provide dedicated youth support workers or provide liason between pediatric and adult support groups.

Where should transition take place?

Transition models include a single step model from a paediatric to and adult clinic or have an intermediary step of either a transition clinic, or a specific adolescent clinic or indeed have two intermediary steps of adolescent clinic to young adult clinic then finally into adult care. Finally where paediatric and adult specialties exist within the same hospital site, transition models can be single site as compared to the more practically challenging split – site models required by stand-alone paediatric hospitals.

Key elements of a transitional care programme

The key elements of successful transitional are a preparation period and education programme for both the young person and their parents. Hospital policies may be age or education based (*i.e.*, at 16 years of age or on completion of secondary or high school), and may need to be reviewed, as rigid enforcement of age-related policies may be detrimental to successful transition for the individual patient. Co-ordination of both transition and eventual transfer is integral to the success of the process as is an interested and capable adult service, willing to continue the transitional process in adult care. Establishing a local network of interested and committed professionals is vital for the success of any transitional care programme. Adequate administrative support for transitional care must not be under-estimated especially in the preparation, updates and distribution of medical summaries to appropriate parties. This in turn facilitates effective communication between all professionals involved in the transition process, integral to successful transition.

It is unlikely that there is a universal transition prescription for all transplant recipients and each is likely to be an individualised plan, which will vary between patients, diseases as well as between centres. Some of the key transitional care issues beyond management of the disease and transplant are discussed below.

Disease education

If the young person has had their primary disease since early childhood, much of the initial disease education may have been primarily directed to the parents. Disease education must be re-taught, acknowledging the changing cognitive development of growing children. The use of age appropriate literature and a skilled play worker or teacher are invaluable to help young people to understand and accept difficult issues such as having a dead person's organ, or facing a life-time of medical monitoring and medication.

One of two requirements for successful transition is an understanding of and an ability of the young person to describe the signs and symptoms requiring urgent medical attention and appropriate literature is vital as well as easy access to medical care, which may be more daunting in an adult unit [7]. Information regarding drugs should extend beyond importance of adherence and side effect profile and monitoring but include rationale, benefits as well as risks, etc.

Generic health education

Generic health issues need to be borne in mind especially as many adult health-promoting behaviours become established during adolescence. Adolescents with chronic illness report more age-related concerns than their healthy peers: acne, alcohol and drug, periods, headaches, anxiety, contraception, insomnia, worry about height and weight and sexual health [8].

- **Sexual health :** in the study mentioned previously, one of the requirements for successful transition is that the young person has an understanding of the implications of the condition and treatments on their sexual and reproductive health [7] as they may be as sexually active as their healthy peers.

It is important to provide information about contraception. Although barrier methods are the safest, there is a high failure rate. It is safe for girls to take a low dose oestrogen/progesterone contraceptive pill or to take the "morning after pill" [8]. Chronic liver disease and/or therapy, however, may cause delayed puberty but this will begin after a successful transplant. Most immunosuppressive drugs are not teratogenic or affect fertility.

Many girls develop menorrhagia post transplant and specific advice from a gyneacologist trained in managing contraception and pregnancy in patients on immunosuppression is particularly useful.

- **Substance misuse :** cigarette smoking has both generic and specific importance with premature arteriosclerosis, hyperlipidaemia, osteoporosis being recognized long-term morbidities of transplantation and simple primary preventive measures should not be ignored. A history of substance misuse has been reported in young people who are non-adherent with medication and hence an important (albeit at times difficult) aspect of history taking [6]. It is important to highlight the importance of sensible behavior, *e.g.*, liver transplant recipients may drink alcohol with their peers in moderation.

- **General exercise :** greater levels of exercise are associated with well-being and long-term functioning in patients with chronic conditions [10] and to be encouraged when feasible, particularly in the light of the concerns of the morbidity of the inactivity of today's youth generally.

Self-advocacy issues

Self-advocacy skills are a key element of transition. Such skills will be useful throughout the lifetime of the individual young person. The focus of self-advocacy skill training is on strengths, capacities and opportunities rather than limitations or deficits, the latter typical of the traditional medical model. Aspects of self-advocacy in the health care include being seen independent from parents by health providers, a full understanding of the illness, involvement in decision-making, self-medication, adherence, etc. The healthcare setting is a safe and often familiar area to practice self-advocacy skills, *e.g.* communication skills, independent living skills, accessing the health service, which are, in turn, important for success in independent living and the world of work.

Seeing the young person independently from the parent helps provide the privacy for such discussions of generic health concerns such as those detailed above, *e.g.* sexual health, alcohol use, with the assurance of confidentiality. In a study of adolescents in primary care, confidentiality was their major priority when surveyed as to the most important attributes of an adolescent friendly practice [11].

Finally, anyone who cares for adolescents should be aware of the legislation of decision-making in this age group in their country. One should always aim for parallel consent, *i.e.* consent from both young person and parent/guardian, even when the young person can consent without parental consent during adolescence. Early involvement in decision-making is important for all young people with a chronic illness and/or disability and simple acknowledgements of this, *e.g.* co-signing consent forms for surgical procedures, etc. are important messages for both the young person and their parents.

Other psychosocial issues

Coping with teasing and/or bullying as well as disclosure issues are important issues to address with the young person during adolescence and transition. Transplant recipients may be particularly vulnerable because of their altered appearance from disease or medication, or because of time lost from school. Disclosure is an important life-long issue whether it refers to disclosing details of the chronic condition and/or therapy to a friend, significant other, potential employer, etc. Exploring and developing coping strategies for disclosure with a health professional can help the young person gain in confidence in this arena.

Vocational issues

Despite the tremendous success story of transplantation in terms of life expectancy, lower levels of employment have been reported in, *e.g.*, adult survivors of a paediatric dialysis and transplant programme [12]. Unemployment was associated with lower educational performance which in turn has been reported to be related to poorer self-esteem [13]. Prospective studies are needed to determine the aetiology of unemployment in young people following transplantation.

Asking a young person with a transplant, what they would like to do when they leave school is therefore an important message, however vague the answer. It is a message that conveys a future beyond the paediatric clinic.

Independence in daily living

The first "work" experiences of children are often within the context of the family with household chores. Being able to drive a car enhances a young person's independence. In the UK, certain young people in receipt of high-level disability living allowance can learn to drive at age 16, one year before their healthy peers. Independence in managing their illness should be fostered from an early age. Many voluntary organisation provide log-books or folders for young people to record health information or medication changes. There are now electronic gadgets to remind patients of the timing of medication as well as recording compliance.

Adherence issues

In any discussion regarding non-adherence in adolescent, it is important to reflect on what young people with chronic diseases have to face day-to-day. They often face long-term therapeutic regimens. They often have to continue medication even when they feel well.

Many drug regimens also required regular monitoring in accordance with the course of the disease. All of these factors potentially lead to restrictions on leisure time, personal freedom, spontaneity and peer interactions. Non-adherent behaviour may be the only control mechanism open to the young person and/or be a simple wish to be heard and to take an active role in the decision making process.

Self-medication is an important aspect of becoming an independent young adult but it must be seen in the context of shared decision-making, self-care and self-management [14]. Experimentation is a normal task of adolescent development and may be practiced by the self-medicating adolescent but in the post-transplantation period non-adherence can be associated with morbidity and even mortality of transplant recipients [15, 16), particularly of late graft loss [17].

It is important to decriminalise non-adherence in the clinic setting and rather than asking "have you been taking your tablets every day", ask "when was the last time you forgot to take your medication".

Peer support

Conventional approaches to promote emotional well-being in young people with chronic illness and/or disability often include referral to psychology services. Peer support may be another means of promoting well-being for such young people. Peer – led programmes in school sex education have been reported to produce behavioural changes that lead to health benefit [18]. Peer education programmes within the context of transplantation programmes may also have similar benefit.

Potential barriers to successful transition

Various barriers to transition can be identified.

The young person

The young person may have a long and close relationship with the paediatric team since disease onset, with whom they saw through their transplant and which they are reluctant to let go of. They may feel safe with the familiar and scared of the unknown – a new hospital, a new team, etc. This is only accentuated by virtue of often unpredictable, uncertain conditions. These young people may also be less mature than their peers, more dependent on their parents and be non-adherent with their therapy. They may still have "paediatric" medical problems such as pubertal delay and growth retardation, the management of which may be unfamiliar to adult teams, never mind their primary diagnoses.

The family of the young person

Likewise the family of the young person may have a similarly close relationship with the pediatric team with little confidence in the adult team and may not understand the importance of age appropriate care for adults. The family may be over-protective of their dependent young person and may resist the attempts of the health-care team to enhance the self-advocacy of their child if not adequately prepared. Their own negative personal experiences of adult healthcare may also make them reluctant to leave the paediatric healthcare team.

The paediatric team

The paediatric team may also not be confident in the adult team in the management of conditions that have important differences from their adult counterparts. They too may rather enjoy the comfort of long-term clinic attendees and postpone the transition and transfer process! The paediatric team must acknowledge the potential intensity of relationships in paediatrics and facilitate the farewell process when the young person eventually transfers to adult care as difficulties in this process can make it difficult for the young person to build new relationships and establish trust in the adult sector.

The adult team

There may be no experienced adult team in late effects of transplantation in childhood or the adult team may indeed have no confidence or training in looking after childhood onset and/or congenital disease. They may assume such diseases are the same as their adult counterparts and forget both the differences in disease manifestations and impact of childhood onset disease. They may also feel that paediatric care is too paternalistic, have higher expectations for learning, personal choice, self-care and independent follow-up and be reluctant to acknowledge the process of transition. They may be less interdisciplinary and more fragmented than their paediatric counterparts. Many young adults find it difficult to make a relationship with the new team and fail to attend regularly. Shared clinics and young adult clinics are important in ensuring smooth transition.

Other barriers

Barriers of lack of planning, time, and geography can also not be ignored. Many "so-called" adolescent issues are true for all ages however, *e.g.* involvement in decision-making, disease education, independence, etc. Differences in delivery must be acknowledged, *e.g.* variations in team working between units. Time allocation for outpatient visits and continuity of professionals between hospital visits may vary between paediatric and adult units. The young person and their families need to be informed of these differences and acquire the skills to negotiate the transfer as well as on-going adult care. A visit of the adult unit and/or a key liaison member of staff are useful in this regard.

Practical issues

Many of the above issues can be overcome by establishing a transition process which includes:

– the development of adolescent facilities including an adolescent clinic with appropriate youth workers, availability of health promotion leaflets;

- ability to see the clinician on their own to discuss intimate problems;
- involvement of the young person in planning their process;
- a "handover clinic or clinics" with the adult unit;
- appointment of a key worker to oversee transition.

The future

Much of the progress in transitional care has been made in the world of paediatric and adolescent health. We now need comparable development at the adult-oriented end of the continuum so that adult-oriented health care is as desirable as what the young person has experienced during childhood, so that transition becomes the normal, expected, planned and desired outcome of paediatric care. Transitional care in the field of transplantation is an area ripe for further research. Close collaboration of professionals working in paediatrics, adolescent health and adult medicine with these young people as well as those with other chronic conditions will hopefully help provide an evidence base for the answers to these questions in the future.

References

1. Blum RW, Garell D, Hadgman CH, et al. Transition from child-centred to adult health-care systems for adolescents with chronic conditions. A position paper of the Society for Adolescent Medicine. *J Adol Health* 1993; 14: 570-6.
2. Mithoefer AB, Supran S, Freeman RB. Risk factors associated with the development of skin cancer after liver transplantation. *Liver Transplant* 2002; 8: 939-44.
3. Ghosh S, Drummond H, Ferguson A. Neglect of growth and development in the clinical monitoring of children and teenagers with inflammatory bowel disease: review of case records. *Br Med J* 1998; 317: 120-1.
4. Sanci LA, Coffey CM, Veit FC, Carr-Gregg M, Patton GC, Day N, Bowes G. Evaluation of the effectiveness of an educational intervention for general practitioners in adolescent health care: randomised controlled trial. *Br Med J* 2000; 320: 224-30.
5. Patterson J, Blum RJ. Risk and resilience among children and youth with disabilities. *Arch Pediatr Adol Med* 1996; 150: 692-8.
6. Lurie S, Shemesh E, Sheiner PA, Emre S, Tindle HL, Melchionna L, Shneider BL. Non-adherence in pediatric liver tranplant recipients – an assessment if risk factors and natural history. *Pediatr Transplant* 2000; 4 (3): 200-6.
7. Scal P, Evans T, Blozis S, Okinow N, Blum R. Trends in transition from pediatric to adult health care services for young adults with chronic conditions. *J Adol Health* 1999; 24: 259-64.
8. Carroll G, Massarelli E, Opzoomer A, Pekeles G, Pedneault M, Frappier JY, Onetto N. Adolescents with chronic disease: are they receiving comprehensive health care? *J Adol Health Care* 1983; 17: 32-6.
9. Sucato G, Murray P. Gynecologic issues of the adolescent female solid organ transplant recipient. *Pediatr Clin North Am* 2003; 50: 1521-42.
10. Stewart AL, Hays RD, Wells KB, Rogers WH, Spritzer KL, Greenfield S. Long-term functioning and well-being outcomes associated with physical activitiy and exercise in patients with chronic conditions in the Medical outcomes study. *J Clin Epidemiol* 1994; 47: 719-30.

11. Croft CA, Asmussen L. A developmental approach to sexuality education: implications for medical practice. *J Adol Health* 1993; 14: 109-14.
12. Reynolds JM, Morton MJ, Garralda ME, Postlethwaite RJ, Goh D. Psychosocial adjustment of adult survivors of a paediatric dialysis and transplant programme. *Arch Dis Child* 1993; 68: 104-10.
13. Morton MJ, Reynolds JM, Garralda ME, Postlethwaite RJ, Goh D. Psychiatric adjustment in end-stage renal disease. A follow-up study of former paediatric patients. *J Psychosomatic Res* 1994; 38: 293-303.
14. Tomlin S. Pharmaceutical care: Improving practice for children in hospital. *Paediatric Nursing* 2001; 13 (4): 25-9.
15. Molmenti E, Mazariegos G, Bueno T. Noncompliance after paediatric liver transplantation. *Trans Proc* 1999; 31: 408.
16. Watson AR. Non-compliance and transfer from paediatric to adult transplant unit. *Pediatr Nephrology* 2000; 14 (6): 469-72.
17. Sudan D. Causes of Late Mortality in pediatric liver transplant. *Ann Surg* 1998; 227: 289-95.
18. Mellanby AR, Phelps FA, Crichton NJ, Tripp JH. School sex education: an experimental programme with educational and medical benefit. *Br Med J* 1995; 311: 414-7.

The IBD patient: transition from childhood to adulthood

Jan Björk

Department of Gastroenterology and Hepatology, Karolinska University Hospital, Stockholm, Sweden

Transferring an adolescent patient to a gastroenterologist requires an understanding of the specific issues and challenges involved in management of pediatric patients with inflammatory bowel disease (IBD).

Epidemiology

In Western World, the incidence of IBD in childhood is 2-5 cases / 100,000 persons / year and the prevalence approximately 20 cases / 100 000 persons. About 10% of the children are diagnosed before 10 years of age, 30% between 11-15 years, and 60% between 16-21 years of age. Crohn's disease (CD) is approximately twice as common as ulcerative colitis (UC) in children and adolescents [1]. In parallel with the trends in the adult IBD population, the incidence of pediatric UC has remained stable, whereas that of pediatric CD has increased in recent decades [2]. In comparison to adult-onset UC, pediatric UC is more often extensive [3].

Genetics

As a clinician who cares for patients with IBD you have several reasons for genetic testing such as predicting susceptibility to disease, disease course, and response to treatment. Appropriate knowledge about the inheritance of IBD is of great importance to be able to give correct information to the adolescent patient and especially to the young adult who considers to become a parent.

Identification of the CARD15/NOD2 gene was a promising step in the direction towards genetic testing [4, 5]. However, the high frequency of CARD15/NOD2 mutations (10-15%) in the normal population (low specificity) combined with the relative infrequency in CD (32.5-46%) (low sensitivity) makes the use of genetic testing impractical for the diagnosis of CD. The genotype-phenotype correlation seen is that CD patients with CARD15/NOD2 mutations have a slightly younger age at onset, as well as more frequent ileal involvement and fibrostenotic disease [6-9]. Testing of unaffected relatives of patients with CD to rule out whether they carry disease-susceptibility mutations is not yet advisable. Such procedure would only be useful if one could counsel the relatives appropriately with respect to their absolute risk of developing CD and eventually provide strategies to prevent or modify disease development. At present, knowledge of family history and ethnical background guides the discussion of CD susceptibility. The frequency of CARD15/NOD2 mutations does not differ between familial and sporadic CD cases; if these mutations were responsible for the CD trait in affected families, one would expect a higher frequency of mutations in familial cases than in sporadic ones. These data indicate that additional genes probably are involved. The estimated relative risk of developing CD based on CARD15/NOD2 genotyping is 1.6-2.78 for a single mutation and 13.63-19 for two mutations in this particular gene [10, 11]. Mutations are equally prevalent in unaffected relatives, but it remains to be seen if they remain asymptomatic over time. A first-degree relative, like a child, of an affected parent has a 5-10 times increased risk to develop CD over time. Another observation is that children tend to be diagnosed with IBD at a younger age than their parents but it is unclear if this represents true genetic anticipation [12, 13]. The frequency of positive family history seems to be higher in children presenting with symptoms before the age of 11 years [14].

Clinical features

As in adults the most common symptoms in UC are frequent bowel movements with bloody and loose stools whereas CD can present itself with a variety of symptoms. At diagnosis, the most common symptom of CD is weight loss, which occurs in 90% of children, followed by diarrhea and abdominal pain. Rectal bleeding and fever are less common and occurs in 20-25% of the children. Like adults, children with IBD may suffer from extraintestinal manifestations where arthritis is the most common manifestation and may precede the onset of bowel symptoms. Other extraintestinal manifestations are erythema nodosum, pyoderma gangrenosum, iritis, episcleritis, uveitis, and primary sclerosing cholangitis (PSC). PSC diagnosed in childhood significantly decreases survival. In a study conducted on 52 children and adolescents, 11 patients underwent liver transplantation and one died during follow-up [15]. Children with IBD are also at an increased risk of thromboembolic complications because of hypercoaguability. The risk of developing extraintestinal manifestation seems to be higher in patients with an onset of CD before the age of 10 years [16]. Linear growth retardation is one of the most troublesome effects of CD. About one third of adult patients with an onset of CD in childhood have a permanent deficit in height [17-20]. A proportion of UC patients with childhood onset of disease also show a deficit in height as adults but this fraction is much smaller than in CD. The degree of growth failure correlates with the severity of intestinal inflammation [21]. Decreased bone mineral density and increased risk of fractures have been reported in children with

IBD [22]. Corticosteroids may exacerbate growth failure and impair bone mineralization emphasising the importance of being aware of the latter complication, especially in young adults with IBD who have been on corticosteroids as children.

Treatment

Corticosteroids

Corticosteroids have long been a mainstay of therapy in CD. Because of the frequent occurrence of side effects in patients treated with corticosteroids, of which prednisolone is the one most frequently used, trials has been conducted with theoretically less harmful compounds. Budesonide has low systemic bioavailability because of its first-pass metabolisation in the liver. In a recent study, the effects and side effects of budesonide and prednisolone were compared. Side effects such as moon face and acne were significantly less frequent in the budesonid group, but remission was obtained more often in prednisolone treated patients after eight weeks although the difference was not significant [23].

Immunomodulatory agents

The use of immunomodulatory therapy including thioguanine compounds (6-mercaptopurine, azathioprine) and metotrexate for IBD in children and adolescents has increased during the last decade. Severe side effects of corticosteroids, like growth suppression, cataracts, glaucoma, osteonecrosis, vertebral collapse, myopathy, and depression is the most important reason for the increased use of such agents. Another important reason is the frequent occurrence of undesirable cosmetic side effects (facial puffiness, hirsutism, weight gain, striae, and acne) which may severely limit their acceptance, especially in teenagers. Bearing this in mind, is it of great importance that the gastroenterologist is fully informed about previous medication, and in patients who have been on corticosteroids for long periods try hard to avoid further use by favouring other treatments. Another important aspect is that knowledge about earlier medical history may help to understand why some young adults who have experienced cosmetic side effects of corticosteroids are hesitant or have a very negative attitude towards these drugs. Nowadays children with moderate to severe IBD are often on azathioprine as maintenance therapy. Even on high-dose treatment severe adverse effects are uncommon. In a study conducted by Fuentes and co-workers only two out of 107 children on azathioprine 3 mg/kg discontinued treatment because of persistent adverse events [24]. Another reason for the increased use of immunomodulatory agents for the treatment of children with IBD is, a change in attitude. This concern regarding risk of malignancy, teratogenicity, and infertility has decreased, whereas the concern for bone marrow and immune suppression remains. Moreover, physicians seem to favour use of immunomodulatory agents over colectomy for children with intractable colitis [25].

Biologic agents

One of the most recent advances in the treatment of CD has been infliximab, a human – murine chimeric antibody to tumor necrosis factor alpha (TNF-α), a proinflammatory cytokine. Applications both in children and adults are corticosteroid dependence, severe corticosteroid side effects and refractivity to, or complications from standard immunosuppressive therapy. The initial clinical response in children with CD is in the range of 60-100% [26-29] but the true sustained response and clinical remission rate will need to be determined by further studies. Moreover, adverse effects have been reported in 3-39% of pediatric patients [30-35]. The prevalence of human antichimeric antibodies (HACA) in children and young adults was about 35% in one study. However, the interval between infusions did not influence the development of HACA and immunomodulatory agents seemed to have a protective role against the development of these antibodies [36].

The treatment is also costly and since the use of infliximab has increased dramatically in the last years and children are receiving continuous treatment with multiple infusions on a regular or on demand basis to be kept in remission. Thus, this is a "problem" that the gastroenterologist has to take over once the patient becomes an adult. The experience from adult patient starting infliximab treatment is that they are very reluctant to discontinue the treatment.

Surgery

Surgery is common in adult patients with CD. Over extended periods of observation the rate of surgery for CD is as high as 80% [37]. Early surgery after diagnosis of disease is also common. In a present study on Crohn patients, 20% were operated upon within three years after diagnosis. In contrast, in a Swedish study on 102 children in northern Stockholm diagnosed with CD between 1990 and 2001, only ten patients underwent surgery and of the 45 UC patients none was operated [2]. This indicates that the need for surgery is less in pediatric and adolescent patients compared to adult patients with IBD. The frequent use of immunomodulatory agents from onset of IBD may contribute to the low frequency of surgery in the pediatric population.

Psychosocial factors

Later in life, when the patient becomes a parent, there are certain circumstances, both positive and negative, that have to be kept in mind. Several studies have shown that parents with IBD develop a closer relationship with their children. On the other hand, parents with symptomatic IBD may have difficulties in caring, especially for young children, a situation which causes worry and guilt in parents. Children reacting with anxiety is not uncommon when the parent is ill or hospitalized, and reactions like anger and frustration to restrictions in social activities are also common, emphasizing that health professionals have an important role to play to provide support for the parent and their children with IBD, and especially for mothers with limited help for their children [38, 39].

Quality in life in children and adolescents with IBD has been estimated by looking at health-related quality of life (HRQoL) using two different questionnaires. Children (8-12 years) were almost comparable with a reference population while adolescents (13-18 years) with IBD had more body complaints and motor dysfunction as well as less autonomy and more negative emotions than the reference population. The impaired motor function and autonomy might make it more difficult to gain independence from caregivers and a high occurrence of negative emotions places adolescents with IBD at risk for depressive and behavioural disorders [40, 41].

Poor compliance can be a problem with severe consequences in adolescent IBD patients, something which may be even more pronounced as the patient becomes an adult. Several reasons can be pointed out. Reluctance to treatment has already been mentioned. Experiences during the course of the disease as a child and adolescent, and family situation must also be taken into consideration. Change to new and unknown health professionals, and decreased support from the parents are other factors of importance. A way to overcome or at least minimize these problems would be to be introduced to the gastroenterologist gradually, starting already in the adolescent phase of the disease.

References

1. Kay M, Wyllie R. The real cost of pediatric Crohn's disease: the role of infliximab in the treatment of pediatric IBD. *Am J Gastroenterol* 2003; 98: 717-20.
2. Hildebrand H, Finkel Y, Grahnquist L, *et al*. Changing pattern of paediatric inflammatory bowel disease in northern Stockholm 1990-2001. *Gut* 2003; 52: 1432-4.
3. Griffiths AM. Specificities of inflammatory bowel disease in childhood. *Best Pract Clin Gastroenterol* 2004; 18: 509-23.
4. Hugot JP, Chamaillard M, Zouali H, *et al*. Association of NOD2 leucine-rich repeat variants with susceptibility to Crohn's disease. *Nature* 2001; 411: 599-603.
5. Ogura Y, Bonen DK, Inohara N, *et al*. A frameshift mutation in NOD2 associated with susceptibility to Crohn's disease. *Nature* 2001; 411: 603-6.
6. Lesage S, Zouali H, Cezard JP, *et al*. CARD15/NOD2 Mutational analysis and genotype-phenotype correlation in 612 patients with inflammatory bowel disease. *Am J Hum Genet* 2002; 70: 845-57.
7. Hampe J, Grebe J, Nikolaus S, *et al*. Association of NOD2 (CARD 15) genotype with clinical course of Crohn's disease: A cohort study. *Lancet* 2002; 359: 1661-5.
8. Cuthbert AP, Fisher SA, Mirza MM, *et al*. The contribution of NOD2 gene mutations to the risk and site of disease in inflammatory bowel disease. *Gastroenterology* 2002; 122: 867-74.
9. Abreu MT, Taylor KD, Lin YC, *et al*. Mutations in NOD2 are associated with fibrostenosing disease in patients with Crohn's disease. *Gastroenterology* 2002; 123: 679-88.
10. Esters N, Pierik M, Steen KV, *et al*. Transmission of CARD15 (NOD2) variants within families of patients with inflammatory bowel disease. *Am J Gastroenterol* 2004; 99: 299-305.
11. Newman B, Silverberg MS, Gu X, *et al*. CARD15 and HLA DRB1 alleles influence susceptibility and disease localization in Crohn's disease. *Am J Gastroenterol* 2004; 99: 306-15.
12. Russell RK, Satsangi J. IBD: a family affair. *Best Pract Res Clin Gastroenterol* 2004; 18: 525-39.
13. Faybush EM, Blanchard JF, Rawsthorne P, Bernstein CN. Generational differences in the age at diagnosis with Ibd: genetic anticipation, bias, or temporal effects. *Am J Gastroenterol* 2002; 97: 636-40.
14. Weinstein TA, Levine M, Pettei MJ, *et al*. Age and family history at presentation of pediatric inflammatory bowel disease. *J Pediatr Gastroenterol Nutr* 2003; 37: 609-13.
15. Feldstein AE, Perrault J, El-Youssif M, *et al*. Primary sclerosing cholangitis in children: a long-term follow-up study. *Hepatology* 2003; 38: 210-7.
16. Gryboski JD. Crohn's disease in children 10 years old and younger: Comparison with ulcerative colitis. *J Pediatr Gastroenterol Nutr* 1994; 18: 174-82.

17. Michener WM, Caulfield M, Wyllie R, Farmer RG. Management of inflammatory bowel disease: 30 years of observation [published erratum appears in *Clev Clin J Med* 1991; 58: 190]. *Clev Clin J Med* 1990; 57: 685-91.
18. Kirschner BS. Growth and development in chronic inflammatory bowel disease. *Acta Paediatr Scand* 1990; 366 (Suppl.): 98-104.
19. Markowitz J, Grancher K, Rosa J, et al. Growth failure in pediatric inflammatory bowel disease. *J Pediatr Gastroenterol Nutr* 1993; 16: 373-80.
20. Kirschner BS. Permanent growth failure in pediatric inflammatory bowel disease. *J Pediatr Gastroenterol Nutr* 1993; 16: 368-9.
21. Motil KJ, Grand RJ, Davis-Kraft L, et al. Growth failure in children with inflammatory bowel disease: a prospective study. *Gastroenterology* 1993; 105: 681-91.
22. Harpavat M, Keljo DJ. Perspectives on osteoporosis in pediatric inflammatory bowel disease. *Curr Gastroenterol Rep* 2003; 5: 225-32 (Review).
23. Escher JC. European Collaborative Research Group on Budesonide in Paediatric IBD. Budesonide versus prednisolone for the treatment of active Crohn's disease in children: a randomized, double-blind, controlled, multicentre trial. *Eur J Gastroenterol Hepatol* 2004; 16: 47-54.
24. Fuentes D, Torrente F, Keady S, Thirrupathy K, et al. High-dose azathioprine in children with inflammatory bowel disease. *Aliment Pharmacol Ther* 2003; 17: 913-21.
25. Markowitz J, Grancher K, Kohn N, Daum F. Immunomodulatory therapy for pediatric inflammatory bowel disease: changing patterns of use, 1990-2000. *Am J Gastroenterol* 2002; 97: 928-32.
26. Baldassano R, Braegger CP, Escher JC, et al. Infliximab (Remicade) therapy in the treatment of pediatric Crohn's disease. *Am J Gastroenterol* 2003; 98: 833-8.
27. Hyams JS, Markowitz J, Wyllie R. Use of infliximab in the treatment of Crohn's disease in children and adolescents. *J Pediatr* 2000; 137: 192-6.
28. Kugathasan S, Werlin SL, Martinez A., et al. Prolonged duration of response to infliximab in early but not late pediatric Crohn's disease. *Am J Gastroenterol* 2000; 95: 3189-94.
29. Vasiliauskas EA, Thomas DW, Schaffer S, et al. Collaborative experience of open label anti-Tnf chimeric monoclonal antibody Remicade in pediatric patients with refractory Crohn's disease. *Gastroenterology* 1999; 116: A584.
30. Kugathasan S, Levy MB, Saeian K, et al. Infliximab retreatment in adults and children with Crohn's disease: Risk factors for the development of delayed severe systemic reaction. *Am J Gastroenterol* 2002; 97: 1408-14.
31. Diamanti A, Castro M, Papadatou B, et al. Severe anaphylactic reaction to infliximab in pediatric patients with Crohn's disease. *J Pediatr* 2002; 140: 636-7.
32. Kamath B., Mamula P., Baldassano R.N., et al. Listeria meningitis after treatment with infliximab. *J Pediatr Gastroenterol Nutr* 2002; 34: 410-2.
33. Reichardt P, Dahnert I, Tiller G, et al. Possible activation of an intramyocardial inflammatory process (Staphylococcus aureus) after treatment with infliximab in a boy with Crohn's disease. *Eur J Pediatr* 2002; 161: 281-3.
34. Mamula P, Markowitz JE, Brown KA, et al. Infliximab as a novel therapy for pediatric ulcerative colitis. *J Pediatr Gastroenterol Nutr* 2002; 34: 307-11.
35. Vanderhoof JA, Young RJ. Autoimmune enteropathy in a child: Response to infliximab therapy. *J Pediatr Gastroenterol Nutr* 2002; 34: 312-6.
36. Miele E, Markowitz JE, Mamula P, Baldassano RN. Human antichimeric antibody in children and young adults with inflammatory bowel disease receiving infliximab. *J Pediatr Gastroenterol Nutr* 2004; 38: 502-8.
37. Mekhjian HS, Switz DM, Melnyk CS, et al. Clinical features and natural history of Crohn's disease. *Gastroenterology* 1979; 77: 898-906.
38. Mukherjee S, Sloper P, Turnbull A. An insight into the experiences of parents with inflammatory bowel disease. *J Adv Nurs* 2002; 37: 355-63.

39. Mukherjee S, Sloper P, Lewin R. The meaning of parental illness to children: the case of inflammatory bowel disease. *Child Care Health Dev* 2002; 28: 479-85.
40. Loonen HJ, Grootenhuis MA, Last BF, Koopman HM, Derkx HH. Quality of life in paediatric inflammatory bowel disease measured by a generic and a disease-specific questionnaire. *Acta Paediatr* 2002; 91: 348-54.
41. Loonen HJ, Grootenhuis MA, Last BF, *et al*. Measuring quality of life in children with inflammatory bowel disease: the impact-II (NL). *Qual Life Res* 2002; 11: 47-56.

New Developments in the Management of Benign GI Disorders.
D.J. Gouma, G.J. Krejs, G.N. Tytgat, Y. Finkel, eds. John Libbey Eurotext, Paris © 2004, pp. 201-215.

Constipation in childhood*

M.A. Benninga

Department of Paediatric Gastroenterology and Nutrition, G8-260, Emma Children's Hospital /Academic Medical Centre, Amsterdam, The Netherlands

Constipation and the involuntary loss of faeces, encopresis have often been regarded as trivial symptoms, which will eventually disappear. However, they seriously interfere with the social and physical well being of the child. Furthermore, these often frustrating symptoms have great impact on family life, leading to parental frustration, accusation and anger. Both symptoms are not always simple to treat and often require prolonged follow-up. Although our understanding of pathophysiology has grown rapidly in recent decades, the causes and management of constipation in childhood remain obscure.

Definition

One of the major problems in studies concerning the management of childhood constipation is the lack of a generally accepted definition for paediatric constipation. This derives mainly from the fact that constipation is a symptom rather than a disease. Constipation is often differently interpreted by patients and physicians [1]. In children, it is even more difficult to define constipation, because the physician relies upon the interpretation of symptoms as told by the parents [2].

In the last two decades the Iowa-criteria were often used in large randomised controlled trials *(table I)* [3]. These criteria were based on the most common features of childhood constipation, *i.e.* infrequent defecation, large stools, encopresis and faecal impaction found on physical examination. The criteria were straightforward, easy to work with and useful in evaluating endpoints of various treatment regimens. However, they did not include the

---

* **Parts of this review are published in:** Benninga MA, Mearin ML. Hypo motility disorders in childhood. Current concepts and treatment. In: Lanschot JJB, Gouma DJ, Jansen PJM, Pinedo HM, Schouten WR, Tytgat GNJ, eds. *Integrated medical and surgical gastroenterology.* Jones EA Houten: Bohn Stafleu & van Loghum, 2004, in press.

Table I. "The Loening-Baucke criteria" [3]

Paediatric constipation	At least two of the following criteria
	1. Defecation frequency less than 3 times a week
2. Two or more encopresis episodes per week
3. Periodic passage of very large amounts of stool once every 7-30 days
4. A palpable abdominal or rectal mass at physical examination.

(The criterion of a large amount of stool is satisfied if it is estimated to be twice the standard amount of stool, shown in a clay model, or if stools are so large that they clog the toilet.) |

whole spectrum of childhood defecation disorders. In 1999, a first attempt was made to categorize childhood functional gastrointestinal disorders using symptom-based diagnostic criteria, based on the expert opinion of paediatric gastroenterologists and psychologists [4]. These Rome II criteria define defecation disorders in childhood based on a presenting symptom profile and include infant dyschezia, functional constipation, functional retention and functional non-retentive faecal soiling (FNRFS) *(table II)*. However, two recent studies concluded that the current Rome-criteria are too restrictive and excluded too many children with constipation. The next Rome criteria should include the most important feature of constipation, encopresis, which is present in approximately 80% of the patients [5, 6].

The universally accepted definition for encopresis (from *copros*, Greek for stool) is the repeated expulsion of a normal bowel movement, whether involuntary or intentional, in inappropriate places (*e.g.* clothing, floor) in a child at least 4 years of age (or equivalent developmental level) (DSM-IV) [2].

Table II. Childhood functional defecation disorders: ROME II – criteria [4]

	Diagnostic criteria
Infant dyschezia	At least 10 minutes of straining and crying before successful passage of soft stools in an other wise healthy child
Functional constipation	In infants and pre-school children at least 2 weeks of:
1) Scybalous, pebble like, hard stools for a majority of stools; or
2) Firm stools two or less times/week; and
3) No evidence of structural, endocrine, or metabolic disease
Functional faecal retention	From infancy to 16 years old, a history of at least 12 weeks of:
1) Passage of large diameter stools at intervals < 2 times/week
2) Retentive poisturing, avoiding defecation by contracting pelvic floor and gluteal muscles
Functional non-retentive faecal soiling	In children older than 4 years, a history of once a week or more for the preceding 12 weeks of:
(1) Defecation into places and at times inappropriate to the social context;
(2) In the absence of structural or inflammatory disease; and
(3) In the absence of signs of faecal retention

Epidemiology

Population based studies in adults in Western-type societies and in Asia have estimated that approximately 10-20% of otherwise healthy people report one or more symptoms of constipation [7, 8]. Little is known about the prevalence of constipation in developing countries. In children constipation represents the chief complaint in 3% of the outpatient visits and 10% to 25% of paediatric gastroenterology visits [3]. In children with cerebral palsy constipation is reported in even 26%- 74% of children [9]. In the Netherlands 1% of the children in the age range of 0-4 years, but hardly any in the range of 4-15 years visits the general practitioner for complaints of constipation [2]. American and British parents reported constipation in toddlers in respectively 16% and 34% of the children [10]. In contrast to adults, constipation in childhood seems to be more common in boys than in girls (2:1), although a 1:1 ratio is also described [11]. In only 10% of all children with defecation disorders, constipation is part of an organic disorder [4].

Encopresis is reported in 1.5-2.8% of children, older than 4 years. In 10-30% of these children encopresis is not secondary to constipation. In this group of children boys are more likely to experience this frustrating symptom than girls, 9:1 [12].

Physiology of defecation

Normal anorectal function strongly depends on the complex interplay between muscles of the pelvic floor, the autonomic and somatic nervous system and the group of muscles controlling the anal sphincters. Faecal continence is warranted by different mechanisms. Firstly, the caudal end of the rectum is closed by the anal sphincter complex, creating an anal sphincter resting pressure of circa 40 mmHg, which is built up by both the internal (for 85%) and external anal sphincter [13]. This pressure increases by a reflex contraction of the external anal sphincter complex when an acute increase of intra-abdominal pressure occurs, thus counteracting the imminent loss of faeces. This function of the anal sphincter is supported by rectal motility, which is directed to keep the rectum empty, transporting faeces back in sigmoidal direction, thus keeping the faeces separated from the anal canal [14]. A final mechanism taking care for continence is the sensation in the cranial part of the anal sphincter. Triggering of receptors in the anal canal by faeces will result in the sensation of imminent faecal loss, giving the person the ability to prevent this loss of faeces by contracting the pelvic floor muscles. When defecation is not desirable, the external sphincter complex, with the help of the pelvic floor, remains contracted, until (due to rectal compliance) the rectal wall has adapted (distension) to the increased rectal volume.

Defecation is elicited by presence of faecal material in the rectum due to peristaltic propagation. Consequently, sensory stimuli in the anal canal provoke a sudden drop in the tone of the internal anal sphincter. By voluntary control it is decided to start defecation by relaxation of the M puborectalis and the M levator. The distension of the rectum evokes a wave of contractions of the rectum and defecation can be completed by voluntary increase in intra-abdominal pressure. The act of defecation depends on maturational control. This control is a process that can be trained when the child (at 1 year of age) slowly discovers the ability to control its pelvic muscles. Before the age of 4 years, most children acquire autonomy and defecation becomes a private, hardly-thought-about activity [2].

A decline in stool frequency from more than four stools per day during the first week of life to one-twto per day at 4 years of age is observed with a corresponding increase in stool size. Approximately 97% of 1-4 years old children pass stool three times daily to once every other day [15].

Pathophysiology

The pathophysiology underlying functional constipation is undoubtedly multifactorial, and not well understood. Difficulties with defecation can result from abnormal function of the different players involved, including the colon, the rectum and the sphincter complex and not al least the will of the child.

In more than 90% of the children no obvious cause can be identified to explain their constipation. In some babies, an acute episode of constipation may occur associated with a change in diet (*i.e.* human to cow's milk) [16]. In "infant dyschezia", it is speculated that neonates fail to coordinate increased intra-abdominal pressure with relaxation of the pelvic floor [3]. Parents need to be reassured that this condition is part of the child's learning process for which no intervention is indicated.

"Retentive posturing" is probably the major cause for the development and/or persistence of constipation in children [17]. Causes of stool withholding are: i) the previous production of a large, hard stool, ii) anal fissures, iii) primarily behavioural mechanism, iv) not taking time to go to the toilet, v) resistance to go to another toilet than their own. When the child experiences an urge to defecate, the toddler assumes an erect posture and holds the legs stiffly together to forcefully contract the pelvic and gluteal muscles. Consequently the rectum accommodates to its content and the urge to defecate disappears. The retained stools become progressively more difficult to evacuate leading to a vicious circle in which the rectum is increasingly distended by large faecal contents. Finally chronic rectal distension may cause overflow soiling, loss of rectal sensitivity and in the end loss of normal urge to defecate. This aberrant behaviour might lead to the unconscious contraction of the external sphincter during defecation, better known as anal sphincter dyssynergia [18]. Approximately 50% of these children show this abnormal defecation pattern. This paradoxal contraction of the anal sphincter complex was thought to be the major pathophysiological mechanism in childhood constipation. However, normalization of this pattern with biofeedback training did not correlate with success treatment [14, 19].

It is unknown if a long-term delay of defecation results in rectal accumulation of faeces and consequently to possible abnormalities in rectal sensation, compliance and motility. And if impaired rectal sensation is secondary to faecal accumulation or due to primary pathophysiological mechanisms [20, 21].

Finally, an overall delay in colonic transit time, slow transit constipation, objectified by colonic transit time measurements, is described in a minority of children with chronic constipation [22]. This might be due to dysfunctioning of the muscles of the colonic wall (resulting in non-powerful contractions) or to dysfunctioning of the enteric nervous system (resulting in non-coordinated motor activity) [23]. Nevertheless, it might also be possible that this overall delay in colonic transit time is due to massive faecal retention in the rectum, slowing down the whole colonic motility.

Some case control studies have shown an association between decreased fibre intake and constipation in children [24]. In contrast, a Dutch study showed no difference in fibre intake between healthy controls and children with chronic constipation [25].

Clinical presentation

The most important complaints of constipated children are a combination of a low defecation frequency and the involuntary loss of faeces *(table III)* [2]. Encopresis often occurs several times a day and in case of severe constipation with rectal impaction it occurs even at night [22]. Often, once every 7-30 days a very large amount of stool is produced, which may clog the toilet. The evacuation of such a large amount of stool is preceded by an increase of the soiling frequency and complaints of abdominal pain and poor appetite. These symptoms disappear immediately after the production of this large amount of stool. In circa 30% of the constipated children there are complaints of urinary tract infections and enuresis [3]. Most constipated children have abdominal and/or rectal faecal impaction upon physical examination.

Encopresis is a source of considerable embarrassment for the child who must deal with taunting by peers. These children may suffer significant emotional setbacks as a result of this problem with social withdrawal, shame, fear of discovery, loss of self esteem and confidence [26]. Therefore, it is not a surprise that children with constipation and encopresis have significantly more behavioural problems than healthy controls [2]. These behaviour problems are however mild and referral to mental health services is rarely needed. Moreover, behavioural profiles in these children significantly improve after successful treatment [12].

Investigations

A careful medical history together with a thorough physical examination is all that is needed for diagnosis and treatment of most children with constipation. Symptom diaries (for diagnostic evaluation and monitoring treatment); colon transit studies (to confirm the patient's complaints and to assess slow transit and regional delay) and anorectal manometry (to exclude Hirschsprung's disease) are sometimes useful. Recently, MRI of the spine revealed spinal abnormalities in 10% of the children with constipation which disappeared after neurosurgery [27].

Table III. Common clinical presentation of constipation

Feature	Percentage (%)
Soiling/encopresis	75-90
Defecation frequency < 3/wk	75
Large stools	75
Straining during defecation	35
Pain during defecation	50-80
Retentive posturing	35-45
Abdominal pain	10-70
Abdominal distension	20-40
Anorexia	10-25
Vomiting	10
Poor appetite	25
Enuresis/Urinary tract infection	30
"Psychological problems"	20
Physical examination	
Abdominal mass	30-50
Anal prolapse	3
Fissures/haemorrhoids	5-25
Faecal impaction	40-100

Medical history

History taking of a child with constipation starts with questions about the defecation pattern in the first year of life. Attention should be paid to the time after birth of the first bowel movement to discriminate functional constipation from Hirschsprung's disease. Often one elicits a history of constipation beginning when an infant was weaned from breast-feeding to a cow's milk-based infant formula. Subsequently, age of onset of bowel problems, stool frequency, the consistency and size of stools, whether defecation is painful, whether blood has been present on the stool or the toilet paper and retentive posturing are issues to be questioned. Furthermore, information about the encopresis frequency, the time of occurrence (day and/or night) and the situation in which encopresis occurs (behind the computer, during play outside) is of major importance. Other important issues that should be discussed are abdominal pain, loss of appetite, urinary tract problems, neuromuscular development and psychological or behavioural problems. A dietary history, medical treatment and previous treatment strategies in relationship to the defecation problems are important to be discussed. In addition, it is essential to ask for possible major events, such as death in the family, birth of a sibling, school problems and sexual abuse.

Physical examination

Total physical and neurological examination should be performed. Abdominal examination gives information concerning accumulation of gas or faeces. Perianal inspection provides information about: the position of the anus, perianal faeces, redness, fissures, haemorrhoids and scars (sexual abuse). At least one digital examination of the anorectum is recommended [28]. The anorectal digital examination assesses perianal sensation, anal tone, the size of the rectum, the amount and consistency of stool in the rectum and the voluntary contraction and relaxation of the anal sphincter.

Abdominal X-ray and colon transit time studies

A plain abdominal radiograph is not indicated to establish the presence of faecal impaction if the rectal examination reveals the presence of large amounts of stool [29]. However, when there is doubt about whether the patient is constipated, a plain abdominal radiograph might be useful in determining the presence of faecal retention in the child who is obese or refuses a rectal examination, or in whom there are other psychological factors (sexual abuse) that make the rectal examination too traumatic.

Assessment of total and segmental colonic transit time (CTT) using radio-opaque markers more accurately and reliably provides relevant information about colorectal motor function in defecation disorders [30]. The marker technique is used to localize the delay in transit time and is helpful if bowel history is unreliable. In adults as well as in children a good relation is found between symptoms of constipation and colonic transit time (CTT) [31, 32]. According to the Bouchoucha method children ingest a capsule with ten radio-opaque markers on six consecutive days [30]. Subsequently, in the morning an abdominal X-ray films is obtained on day 7. Localization of markers on abdominal films relies on the identification of bony landmarks and gaseous outlines. Segmental transit time is obtained by multiplying the number of markers in the segment of interest.

Studies in adults and children with complaints of constipation show different CTT patterns: i) normal colonic transit time; normal transit time through all colonic segments; ii) outlet obstruction: delayed transit time through the anorectal region and slow transit constipation: prolonged transit time through the entire colon. Normal transit times are measured in about 39% to 58% of the constipated children [29, 36]. The most common type of delayed CTT in children is situated in the rectum, outlet obstruction [29, 33].

Finally, the marker test is useful to differentiate between children with constipation and children with FNRFS. Approximately 90% of the children with FNRFS have a normal CTT and have normal values upon anorectal manometry. A normal CTT in combination with a normal defecation frequency without a rectal mass on physical examination confirms the diagnosis FNRFS [34]. These children are best treated with a strict toilet training program and should not be treated with oral laxatives since it increases the encopresis frequency [35].

Anorectal manometry

Anorectal manometry measures pressures in the anorectal region and provides a way of quantifying the function of the internal and external sphincters. Many investigators have performed these studies, but lack of standardization in methods (open-tipped perfusion, closed triple-balloon, pressure transducers) of performing anorectal manometry has resulted in inconsistencies [2]. Anorectal manometry shows that children with constipation have either impaired rectal sensation, that is, the smallest volume of distension that is sensed by the subject or even have a megarectum [36]. However, compliance of the rectum and the age of the children will significantly influence the threshold for sensation measured as volume. Future studies using pressure-controlled distension will hopefully shed new light on these shortcomings in measuring visceral sensation. Furthermore, manometric studies in these children showed decreased rectal contractility on attempted defecation and paradoxical contraction of the external anal sphincter and puborectal muscles during defecation attempts, also known as anismus or pelvic floor dyssynergia or a combination. Pelvic floor dyssynergia occurs in more than 50% of the constipated children. However, achievement of normalisation of pelvic floor dyssynergia after biofeedback training was not associated with success. Therefore this phenomenon seems not to play a crucial role in the pathogenesis of childhood constipation.

Manometry, however is a good screening test for Hirschsprung's disease. The presence of the anorectal, a relaxation of the internal sphincter induced by transient distension of a rectal balloon, excludes Hirschsprung's disease. It is absent in children with Hirschsprung's disease. Term and premature infants older than 26 weeks' postmenstrual age (PMA) have a normal developed anorectal reflex to rectal distension [37].

Treatment

The oral or rectal laxative treatment of constipation is mainly based on empirical experience, but not on placebo controlled randomised studies [38]. Therefore, the best "evidence-based" treatment cannot be constructed and almost all advices concerning the use of oral or rectal laxatives are based on clinical empirical experience. Only a few randomised studies, most of them with small patient numbers, have been performed evaluating new treatments such as biofeedback training for children with defecation disorders.

The treatment of acute simple constipation consists of dietary advices, filling out a diary and toilet training. The treatment of chronic constipation in childhood is based on four important phases: i) education, ii) disimpaction, iii) prevention of reaccummulation of faeces and iv) follow-up.

It is important to treat constipation early in childhood to prevent development of severe constipation or faecal soiling or both [16]. Large studies in the US and Great Britain showed that constipated children < 2 years of age responded better to treatment than children > 2 years of age.

Treatment of acute simple constipation

Dietary measures

For most infants with acute simple constipation, dietary measures, including an increase in fluid and carbohydrate intake often corrects the problem. Toddlers and older children usually respond to increasing fluids and encouraging increasing dietary fibre intake [24].

Diary

The child, with help of the parents, fills out a diary to objectify complaints, to quantify therapeutic progress and to enhance motivation. This stresses once more that the child is responsible for the defecation problem. The diary card is linked to a rewarding system.

Toilet training

Another simple general measure to normalize defecation is toilet training. At the start of the treatment the child is instructed to attempt to defecate three times a day during five minutes, after the meal. The child is stimulated to strain actively while placing its feet on a foot-rest. The latter is important to flatten the anorectal angle, facilitating faecal expulsion.

Treatment of chronic constipation

Education

The first essential in treatment is to gain the family's confidence and explain the mechanism of the symptoms. It is crucial for both the child and the parent to express that it is nobody's fault, to alleviate guilt, explaining with the help of drawings that soiling is a consequence of the full rectum, and to decrease the feeling of shame. The child and parents almost invariably accept a positive non-accusatory approach with relief. Furthermore, it should be explained that the treatment is often longstanding and marked by periods of improvement alternating with deterioration.

Disimpaction

Treatment of severe faecal impaction in the rectum should begin by administering enemas for three consecutive days before oral laxatives are started [2]. If the rectum is clogged with hard stool, treatment with oral laxatives, without removing these scybala with enema's, will paradoxically result in an increase in soiling due to overflow diarrhoea and an increase in abdominal pain and bloating.

In practice, enemas with lower volume will be prescribed to children less than 10 kg of bodyweight, whereas older children preferentially receive larger volume enemas (sodium-dioctylsulfosuccinate and sorbitol or phosphate-enema) *(table IV)*. If the faecal mass has

Table IV. Frequently used laxatives (dosage and side effects)

Laxative	Dosage	Side effects
Lactulose	1-3 ml/kg 1 or 2 times daily	Flatulence, abdominal pain
Lactitol	5-40 gr/1 or 2 times daily	Flatulence, abdominal pain
Magnesium oxide	500-2000 gr/day	Hypermagnesaemia; due to concurrent renal failure
Milk of Magnesia	> 6 months: 1-3 ml/kg/day (divide into 1-2 doses)	See Magnesium oxide
PEG 3350-4000 Maintenance	0.26-0.84 gr/kg/day	Loose stools, bad taste (PEG + additional electrolytes)
PEG 3350 Disimpaction	1-1.5 gr/kg/day (3 to 4 days)	Loose stools, bloating/flatulence, nausea, vomiting
Mineral oil (liquid paraffin)	> 12 months: 1-3 ml/kg/day (maintenance) Disimpaction: 30 ml/10 kg body weight Or: 15-30 ml orally per year of age per day. Max.: 240 ml 1 or 2 times daily for 3 days	Bad taste, anal leakage, aspiration pneumonia (< 12 months, dysphagia)
Barley Malt extract (Maltsupex)	5-10 ml in 60-120 ml of water/juice 2 times daily (breast fed infants) 2-10 ml per 240 ml of milk/juice (bottle fed infants)	Flatulence, bloating, nausea
Bisacodyl Oral	5 mg every other day-10 mg daily	Abdominal cramps, abdominal pain, diarrhoea
Bisacodyl Rectal	5 mg suppositories (3 days)	Abdominal cramps, anal irritation abdominal pain
Glycerin suppositories	< 6 years: 1 paediatric supp. (1 gr) ≥ 6 years: 1 adult supp. (2 or 3 gr)	Anal irritation
Sodium docusate + sorbitol enema "Klyx"	< 6 year: 60 ml, > 6 years: 120 ml	Abdominal cramps
Sodium bisphosphate enema "Fleet"	> 20 kg, adult size enema	In case of renal problems or M. Hirschsprung: Hyper-phosphataemia, other electrolyte disturbances
Sodiumlaurylsulfo-actetate enema "Microlax"	Infants < 10 kg	Anal irritation
Senna Senokot syrup (granules/tablets)	1-5 years: 5 ml 1 to 2 times daily > 5 years: 10 ml/day	Abdominal cramps, melanosis coli, yellowish-brown urine
Lavage PEG 3350 orally/NG-tube	15.5-183 ml/kg first stool after 2.8 hours 1-1.5 g/kg/day (3 to 4 days) first stool after 1.89 days	Nausea, vomiting, abdominal cramps, pulmonary aspiration/oedema

been removed successfully, but soiling relapses or the defecation frequency does not normalize with adequate treatment with oral laxatives, enemas are added to the long-term treatment. Regular use of enemas is sometimes needed but the effect on long-term administration on the rectal mucosa has never been studied.

For a child who strongly fears enemas, the faecal mass can be softened and liquefied with large quantities of osmotic agents or a polyethylene glycol (PEG) solution. A 3-day administration of PEG 3350 at doses of 1 and 1.5 g/kg was safe and effective in the treatment of severe childhood faecal impaction [39].

Prevention of reaccumulation of faeces

Oral laxatives (table IV)

Once disimpaction has been achieved, it is essential to begin an oral daily laxative immediately and continue this treatment for months or longer if necessary to prevent reaccumulation of retained stools and overcoming stool withholding if present. The correct dose is that which produces a daily soft stool without side effects.

Most times the treatment is started with an osmotic laxative (e.g. lactulose or lactitol) in a dose of 6 gram per kg bodyweight, divided in two portions per day [2]. The main function of the osmotic laxatives is to loosen stool consistency, thus facilitating transport and expulsion and rendering defecation less painful. The dose is increased until improvement is achieved (sometimes up to 2-3 times the starting dose). During the first days flatulence may occur whereas abdominal pain can increase especially on higher doses of laxatives. The dose should be titrated based on the defecation frequency aiming at a frequency of ≥ 3/week. In addition, faecal accumulation in the rectum should be prevented. This adequate dose should be continued for at least three months. Long-term administration in adults appears to have no adverse effects [40]. However, lactulose as monotherapy is often not sufficient and additional medication, such as the stimulant laxative bisacodyl (5-15 mg every other day) might be useful. Good results of the prokinetic cisapride (4 dd 0.2 mg/kg) have been reported in small randomised studies with a significant higher success percentage compared to placebo (76% versus 37%) [41]. However, since serious side effects, such as prolonged QTc-interval, have been described, the use of cisapride in the treatment of childhood constipation is rare. Bisacodyl leads to apoptosis of colonic epithelial cells with accumulation of phagocytic macrophages containing cellular remnants, but these are not pigmented [40]. Apart from these changes, there does not appear to be any evidence that polyphenolic laxatives cause adverse effects on long-term use.

Polyethylene glycol (PEG) is an inert polymer with a range of molecular weight. In the range of 3,200 to 4,000 the compound is not absorbed by the gut and is excreted unchanged in the faeces. The osmotic pressure of PEG in the colon opposes the absorption of water, with the result that the faeces are softened and increased in bulk, or become liquid. PEG 3350 has been shown to be a useful alternative in the treatment of constipation in children [42].

Behavioural therapy

The aim of a combination of behavioural (toilet training in combination with a rewarding system, diminishing of toilet phobia), cognitive (psychotherapy, cognitive and family therapy, or educational intervention) and laxative treatment is to lower the level of distress and develop or restore normal bowel habits by positive reinforcement, preservation of self-respect and encouragement of the child and parents during the treatment. In a small randomised controlled trial a combination of intensive medical therapy and an enhanced toilet training program was significantly more effective than intensive medical treatment alone [43].

Psychological referral is indicated in children who fail intensive medical treatment and in those with severe emotional problems or serious family problems. In these patients it is preferred to combine psychiatric and paediatric treatment strategies.

Biofeedback training

In more than 50% of children with defecation disorders, the external anal sphincter and puborectalis muscle contract instead of relax during defecation. It is possible to normalize this phenomenon with the help of biofeedback training. However, we previously showed that normalisation is not related to successful outcome [18]. Also the improvement of the sensation of urge with this technique did not lead to a higher success rate compared to children receiving only medical therapy. The role of biofeedback training in the treatment of defecation disorders in children seems to be limited.

Surgery

There is no place for anal dilatation and internal sphincterotomy in the treatment of constipation since both techniques have a high risk of faecal incontinence. Endosonography showed damage of the anal sphincter complex in more than 50% of the patients [44].

In patients with severe constipation that leads to hospitalisation, those in whom multiple medical regimens have failed, those who refuse either oral medications or retrograde enemas and those without generalized colonic motility might benefit from antegrade cleaning of the colon. A continent appendicocoecostomia (Malone stoma) through which the cecum can be intermittently catheterised for administration of an antegrade enema proofed to be safe and effective in neurologically intact children with severe constipation [45]. Complications include leakage of the irrigation solution, granulation tissue, and tube dislodgement. Side effects include abdominal cramping and soiling after administration of the antegrade enema.

Follow-up and prognosis

Frequent follow-up in patients with constipation is of major importance since relapse of symptoms occurs in 50% of the children. After three months the laxatives can be reduced provided that a normal bowel habit is maintained. About 50% of the children with chronic constipation require treatment and close follow-up for at least six to twelve months [42].

Follow-up studies in children with constipation show a cure rate of approximately 40% after one year of intensive medical and behavioural treatment [46]. Moreover, long-term follow-up studies even show that after five years of intensive medical and behavioural treatment 50% of children still suffer of constipation and encopresis. A large cohort of 418 Dutch children with constipation older than 5 years at intake (279 boys; median age 8.0 years) was prospectively followed using a standardized questionnaire [47]. Approximately 60% of the patients had achieved success by one year. Despite intensive initial medical and behavioural treatment, 30-50% of these children persist to have severe symptoms of constipation after five years of follow-up and these symptoms are even present beyond 18 years of age. Another important finding was that 50% of the children had at least one relapse within the first five years after initial treatment success, underscoring the need to continue frequent follow-up visits for at least one year after successful treatment to prevent or treat with laxatives a possible relapse.

References

1. Feldman M, Friedman LS, Sleizenger MH. Sleizenger & Fordtran's. *Gastrointestinal and Liver Disease Constipation*. Philadelphia: Saunders, 2002 : 181-210.
2. Benninga MA. *Constipation and faecal incontinence in childhood*. Thesis. Baarn: Bosch en Keuning, 1994.
3. Loening-Baucke V. Chronic constipation in children. *Gastroenterology* 1993; 105: 1557-64.
4. Rasquin-Weber A, Hyman PE, Cucchiara S, Fleisher DR, Hyams JS, Milla, *et al.* Childhood functional gastrointestinal disorders. *Gut* 1999; 45: 60-8.
5. Voskuijl WP, Heijmans J, Heymans HS, Taminiau JA, Benninga MA. The use of Rome II criteria in childhood defecation disorders; Applicability in clinical and research practice. *J Pediatr* 2004, in press.
6. Loening-Baucke V. Functional fecal retention with encopresis in childhood. *J Pediatr Gastroenterol Nutr* 2004; 38: 79-84.
7. Talley NJ, Jones M, Nuyts G, Dubois D. Risk factors for chronic constipation based on a general practice sample. *Am J Gastroenterol* 2003; 98: 1107-11.
8. Cheng C, Chan AO, Hui WM, Lam SK. Coping strategies, illness perception, anxiety and depression of patients with idiopathic constipation: a population-based study. *Aliment Pharmacol Ther* 2003; 18: 319-26.
9. Elawad MA, Sullivan PB. Management of constipation in children with disabilities. *Dev Med Child Neurol* 2001; 43: 829-32.
10. Loening-Baucke, V. Constipation in children. *N Engl J Med* 1998: 339: 1155-8.
11. Van Ginkel R, Büller HA, Boeckxstaens GE, Der Plas RN, Taminiau JA, Benninga MA. The effect of anorectal manometry on the outcome of treatment in severe childhood constipation: a randomized, controlled trial. *Pediatrics* 2001; 108: E9.
12. Van der Plas RN, Benninga MA, Redekop WK, Taminiau JA, Büller HA. Randomised trial of biofeedback training for encopresis. *Arch Dis Child* 1996; 75: 367-74.
13. Speakman CT, Kamm MA. The internal and sphincter: new insights into faecal incontinence. *Gut* 1991; 32: 345-6.
14. Rao SS, Welcher K. Periodic rectal motor activity: the intrinsic colonic gatekeeper? *Am J Gastroenterol* 1996; 91: 890-7.
15. Fontana M, Bowel frequency in healthy children. *Acta Paediatr Scand* 1989; 78: 682-4.
16. Iacono G, Cavataio F, Montalto G, Florena A, Tumminello M, Soresi M, Notabartolo A, Carroccio A. Intolerance of cow's milk and chronic constipation in children. *N Engl J Med* 1998: 339: 1100-4.

17. Loening-Baucke V. Constipation in early childhood: patient characteristics, treatment, and longterm follow-up. *Gut* 1993; 34: 1400-4.
18. Van der Plas RN, Benninga MA, Büller HA, Bossuyt PM, Akkermans LMA, Taminiau JAJM. Biofeedback training in treatment of childhood constipation: a randomised controlled study. *Lancet* 1996; 348: 776-80.
19. Loening-Baucke V. Biofeedback treatment for chronic constipation and encopresis in childhood: long-term outcome. *Pediatrics* 1995; 96: 105-10.
20. Meunier P, Louis D, deBeaujeu MJ. Physiologic investigation of primary chronic constipation in childhood: comparison with the barium enema study. *Gastroenterology* 1984; 87: 1351-7.
21. Van der Plas RN, Benninga MA, Staalman CR, Akkermans LMA, Redekop WK, Taminiau JA, Büller HA. Megarectum in constipation. *Arch Dis Child* 2000; 83: 52-8.
22. Benninga MA, Büller HA, Tytgat GNJ, Akkermans LMA, Bossuyt PM, Taminiau JAJM. Colonic transit time in constipated children; does pediatric slow transit constipation exist? *J Ped Gastroenterol Nutr* 1996; 23: 241-51.
23. Di Lorenzo C, Flores AF, Reddy SN, Hyman PE. Use of colonic manometry to differentiate causes of intractable constipation in children. *J Pediatr* 1992; 120: 690-5.
24. Roma E, Adamidis D, Nikolara R, Constantopoulos A, Messaritakis J. Diet and chronic constipation in children: the role of fiber. *J Ped Gastroenterol Nutr* 1999; 28: 169-74.
25. Mooren GC, van der Plas RN, Bossuyt PM, Taminiau JA, Büller HA. The relationship between intake of dietary fiber and chronic constipation in children. *Ned Tijdschr Geneeskd* 1996; 140: 2036-9.
26. Abrahamian FP, Lloyd-Still JD. Chronic constipation in childhood: a longitudinal study of 186 patients. *J Pediatr Gastroenterol Nutr* 1984; 3: 460-7.
27. Nurko S. Spinal cord abnormalities in children with intractable constipation. *Gastroenterology* 2002: A M1513.
28. Baker SS, Liptak GS, Colletti RB, Croffie JM, Di Lorenzo C, Ector W, Nurko S. Constipation in infants and children: evaluation and treatment. *J Pediatr Gastroenterol Nutr* 1999; 29: 612-26.
29. Benninga MA, Büller HA, Staalman CR, Gubler DF, Bossuyt PM, van der Plas RN, Taminiau JAJM. Defecation disorders in children, colonic transit *versus* the Barr score. *Eur J Pediatr* 1995; 154: 277-84.
30. Bouchoucha M, Devroede G, Arhan P. What is the meaning of colorectal transit measurements? *Dis Colon Rectum* 1992; 35: 773-82.
31. Glia A, Lindberg G, Nilsson LH, Mihocsa L, Akerlund JE. Clinical value of symptom assessment in patients with constipation. *Dis Colon Rectum* 1999; 42: 1401-8.
32. Zaslavsky C, da Silveira TR, Maguilnik I. Total and segmental colonic transit time with radio-opaque markers in adolescents with functional constipation. *J Pediatr Gastroenterol Nutr* 1998; 27: 138-42.
33. Gutierrez C, Marco A, Nogales A, Tebar R Total and segmental colonic transit time and anorectal manometry in children with chronic idiopathic constipation. *J Pediatr Gastroenterol Nutr* 2002; 35: 31-8.
34. Benninga MA, Büller HA, Heymans HS, Tytgat GN, Taminiau JA. Is encopresis always the result of constipation? *Arch Dis Child* 1994; 71: 186-93.
35. Van Ginkel R, Benninga MA, Blommaart PJE, vd Plas RN, Boeckxstaens GE, Büller HA, Taminiau JAJM. Biofeedback training or oral laxatives in functional non-retentive fecal soiling? *J Pediatr* 2000; 137: 808-13.
36. Meunier P, Mollard P, Marechal JM. Physiopathology of megarectum: the association of megarectum with encopresis. *Gut* 1976; 17: 224-7.
37. De Lorijn F, Omari TI, Kok JH, Taminiau JA, Benninga MA. Maturation of the rectoanal inhibitory reflex in very premature infants. *J Pediatr* 2003; 143: 630-3.
38. Price KJ, Elliott TM. What is the Role of Stimulant Laxatives in the Management of Childhood Constipation and Soiling? *Cochrane Database Syst Rev* 2001; 3: CD002040.

39. Youssef NN, Peters JM, Henderson W, Shultz-Peters S, Lockhart DK, Di Lorenzo C. Dose response of PEG 3350 for the treatment of childhood fecal impaction. *J Pediatr* 2002; 141: 410-4.
40. Gattuso JM, Kamm MA. Adverse effects of drugs used in the management of constipation and diarrhoea. *Drug Saf* 1994; 10: 47-65.
41. Nurko S, Garcia-Aranda JA, Worona LB, Zlochisty O. Cisapride for the treatment of constipation in children: A double-blind study. *J Pediatr* 2000; 136: 35-40.
42. Loening-Baucke VA. Polyethylene glycol without electrolytes for children with constipation and encopresis. *J Pediatr Gastroenterol Nutr* 2002; 34: 372-7.
43. Borowitz SM, Cox DJ, Sutphen JL, Kovatchev B. Treatment of childhood encopresis: a randomized trial comparing three treatment protocols. *J Pediatr Gastroenterol Nutr* 2002; 34: 378-84.
44. Nielsen MB, Rasmussen OO, Pedersen JF, Christiansen J. Risk of sphincter damage and anal incontinence after anal dilatation for fissure-in-ano. An endosonographic study. *Dis Colon Rectum* 1993; 36: 677-80.
45. Youssef NN, Barksdale Jr E, Griffiths JM, Flores AF, Di Lorenzo C. Management of intractable constipation with antegrade enemas in neurologically intact children. *J Pediatr Gastroenterol Nutr* 2002; 34: 402-5.
46. Staiano A, Andreotti MR, Greco L, Basile P, Auricchio S. Long-term follow-up of children with chronic idiopathic constipation. *Dig Dis Sci* 1994; 39: 561-4.
47. Van Ginkel R, Reitsma JB, Buller HA, van Wijk MP, Taminiau JA, Benninga MA. Childhood constipation: Longitudinal follow-up beyond puberty. *Gastroenterology* 2003; 125: 357-63.

Achevé d'imprimer par Corlet, Imprimeur, S.A.
14110 Condé-sur-Noireau
N° d'Imprimeur : 78968 - Dépôt légal : septembre 2004

Imprimé en France